THE
LOST VOICE

THE
LOST VOICE

A Memoir

GRETA MORGAN

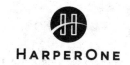

HarperOne

An Imprint of HarperCollins*Publishers*

THE LOST VOICE. Copyright © 2025 by Greta Morgan. All rights reserved. Printed in the United States of America. No part of this book may be used or reproduced in any manner whatsoever without written permission except in the case of brief quotations embodied in critical articles and reviews. For information, address HarperCollins Publishers, 195 Broadway, New York, NY 10007.

HarperCollins books may be purchased for educational, business, or sales promotional use. For information, please email the Special Markets Department at SPsales@harpercollins.com.

FIRST EDITION

Designed by Kyle O'Brien

Library of Congress Cataloging-in-Publication Data has been applied for.

ISBN 978-0-06-341196-8

25 26 27 28 29 LBC 5 4 3 2 1

For Mom, Dad, and Garrett.
For everyone who listens.

Since my house burned down / I now own a better view / of the rising moon

—Mizuta Masahide

CONTENTS

ONE

SOMETHING IS WRONG

YOU NEVER KNOW WHEN IT'S THE LAST TIME. THERE WAS A LAST time that I crawled, a last time I used training wheels on my bike, a last night that my immediate family lived under one roof. There were last kisses in fading relationships, last shows with bands that broke up, last laughs with friends who have died. One day, I'll climb a mountain for the last time, talk to my parents for the last time, see a sunset for the last time.

My singing voice was as constant as my heartbeat, as unique as my fingerprints, as necessary to my self-recognition as seeing my face in the mirror. Despite this awareness of life's endings, I somehow never expected that there would be a *last time* that I would sing with my steady, reliable voice.

In September 2019, Vampire Weekend sold out Madison Square Garden. Since joining the touring band a year earlier, I had played synthesizer, piano, guitar, and percussion, sometimes all of them within one song. Walking onto the stage that night felt like entering a pulsing city made of amps and cables and speakers; electricity sizzling through every wire. The hum of the arena reminded me of summer nights when the air vibrates, just before lightning strikes.

I stood stage left, in the back row, with two keyboards in front of me and a half circle of guitars standing behind me. I was wearing a bright orange tracksuit with shorts and white suede sneakers. Before the show, one of my bandmates joked that I was the missing Spice Girl—Pumpkin Spice. In the middle of the set, we sang "New Dorp. New York" and I played a six-inch cylindrical shaker with my left hand for eleven minutes straight; I called it "the eleven-minute hand job."

As we hit the dance bridge, MSG lit up like a giant red galaxy; the audience wore light-up wristbands synced to our stage lights. Our drummer pounded the kick drum, *thumTHUM thumTHUM*, like a heartbeat, my own heart pounding as I anticipated what was coming next. He hit the cymbal crash to end the song and the stage lights went dark.

My legs trembled, but they carried me center stage. The adrenaline running through my body felt like a swarm of bees. My eyes were closed when the spotlight found me, turning my eyelids a peachy pink. The crowd thundered with applause when they noticed that the only woman in the band was now at the microphone. Our guitarist fingerpicked the opening riff and the first phrase of the song came out of my mouth. *I know the reason why you think I oughta stay . . .*

My voice rose from a small place inside me and filled the

entire arena. The sound surrounded me like a warm bath, my voice the fountain from which it poured. Performing felt effortless, easier than speaking. Ezra, our lead singer, had written the song, but I found an emotional entry into it as if it were one of my own.

I know the reason why you think I oughta stay
funny how you're telling me on my wedding day . . .

I sang it from the tender spot in my heart that remembered the love that had slipped from my hands. The kind of love that felt like finding a paradise island, but then losing the coordinates forever. I inhabited the words like a method actor, willing them to feel true. Singing that night felt like summiting the highest peak of my voice, after a lifetime of climbing.

Have you ever seen a bird ride a wave of wind, coasting across the whole sky without flapping its wings? That was how this felt. Soaring, but my feet were on the ground. When the last word of the chorus rose from my mouth, the crowd roared with applause, the high-pitched cheers of women's voices cutting through the most. I opened my eyes, and even though I couldn't see the exact faces of the thousands and thousands of people out there clearly, I could sense them smiling at me. "Greta Morgan, everyone," Ezra said into the microphone, then motioned for applause.

At the after-party, two of my old Chicago friends, Bobby and Deidre, sandwiched me in a hug. "Gretzky! You killed it!" Bobby said. We'd been friends ever since he played a few shows in one of my former bands, Gold Motel, in 2010. "Do you remember when we played the Frog Bar in Cleveland for, like, eleven people?" he asked. "And weren't five of them in the opening band?"

"Don't remind me," I said, laughing. It had been nine years since then—when I was twenty-one. After that show, the promoter had held the $400 guarantee in his grip, seemingly reluctant to hand it over. "I expected you to bring a bigger crowd," he had said, letting out an exhausted sigh.

Like a good Midwesterner, I reflected the attention back onto my friends. "Tell me about the move to New York," I said to Bobby and Deidre now. "How are you all liking it so far?"

"Not so fast," Deidre said. She put her hands on my shoulders and shook me like she was trying to bring me back to my senses. "Greta, are you celebrating this?" she said. "You worked your *entire life* for this and you fucking got it." I *was* celebrating. When I started my first band, The Hush Sound, in my mom's basement, at age fifteen, I never imagined I would one day sing on the same stage where my idols—Joni Mitchell, Nina Simone, Bruce Springsteen, Simon and Garfunkel, George Harrison, Bob Dylan, and the Beach Boys—had once performed.

Still, this wasn't *exactly* what I'd worked my entire life for. Being a touring musician in one of my favorite bands was a once-in-a-lifetime job, of course, but my truest passion was songwriting, and the Vampire Weekend records had none of my creative input. Danielle Haim had recorded the lead vocals on "Hold You Now," the song I'd just sung at Madison Square

4

Garden. Her voice is rich, deep, and earthy, and she performed the song with a guttural kind of punctuation. During rehearsals, the band encouraged me to sing it the way Danielle had.

When I made my own records, what mattered was that my voice sounded original, that it felt like me, and that it could clearly express the truth of my inner world. Once I joined Vampire Weekend, what mattered was my malleability, my ability to blend into a layered choir of backing *ahhhhhs* or the imitation of the female lead vocals on the record. After the album cycle ended, I'd return to performing my own songs. The highs of sold-out Vampire Weekend shows had satisfied a lifelong dream of performing for huge crowds, but they also ignited a hunger to grow my solo career.

My first band, The Hush Sound, had a wild streak of beginner's luck. After our first album was released in 2005, we were signed to a major label and I soon went on my first arena tour opening for Fall Out Boy, all while finishing my senior year of high school by correspondence. When we started the band, I was a sophomore in Catholic school and my voice sounded as delicate and innocent as I was.

Over the next fifteen years, I made eight records with three bands, played hundreds of concerts, and grew from a shy fifteen-year-old girl to a self-assured thirty-year-old woman. When I started The Hush Sound, I wrote slow and simple melodies to suit my limited vocal range and dynamics. My gentle folk ballads were built around lilting classical piano and dreamy imagery to carry the emotional power. My bandmates arranged the songs, and producers built the sonic landscapes of our records.

But on *Midnight Room*, my last full-length record made as a solo project, my songwriting had blossomed. I belted out huge choruses, played many of the instruments on the record, created sprawling soundscapes, and discovered a breadth of musical expression I never knew I had.

I was excited for the next phase. At thirty-one, I'd fully cultivated my musical powers and felt ready to make the most distinct, truest record ever. I had admired Bobbie Gentry, Dusty Springfield, Linda Ronstadt, and Roberta Flack for their sultry, rich, nuanced voices. I wanted to make a record that spotlighted my voice, using piano as the backbone and building lush orchestrations around it. Till this point, most of my songs masked the truth in poetic ambiguity. But I admired the way country songwriters could capture a film's worth of narrative in the length of a song. I wondered whether it might be possible to combine that level of storytelling with cinematic, sunshine-y, dream-pop. I longed to write songs with clearer stories, with bigger choruses, than I'd ever written before.

After the after-party, there was an after-after-party at a loft in Midtown. The speakers were blasting so loudly that I practically had to scream to be heard. When I couldn't stand any longer, my body exhausted and senses fried, our day-to-day manager walked me back to the hotel. When I staggered into my room after 3 a.m., my mind was still buzzing with an adrenaline afterglow, but my body was so tired that it felt like my limbs were made of wet concrete. I washed my makeup off, undressed, and crawled into bed. I scrolled some videos that people had shared from the show on social media. Seeing myself sing center stage at Madison Square Garden was surreal—this was one of the exact fantasies I'd longed to create ever since I was a kid.

I turned on the noisemaker next to the bed and electronic crickets chirped loud enough to drown out the street sounds below—almost. My Little Martin acoustic guitar always slept beside me on tour, its headstock on the pillow, its body parallel to mine. I reached for him, held him against my chest, and hummed the new song I had started writing earlier that morning:

> *Woke up in a cold sweat*
> *From a dream I don't understand yet*
> *I was the last person on earth . . .*
> *With one of every color of paint*
> *I went to the streets to graffiti names*
> *I painted yours in baby blue . . .*

The song was arriving in fragments, but the chorus hadn't crystallized yet. Like watching a camera viewfinder turning from blur into focus, the song became clearer each time I sat down to write.

On the verge of sleep, I relived the show. In my mind's eye, I was center stage again, this time wearing a floor-length blue silk dress like the one Joni Mitchell had worn at Carnegie Hall in 1972. I was the version of myself one evolution ahead, more graceful, more confident, thinner, with an even more dynamic voice. When the spotlight lit me with the warm golden glow, out came *my* song, the one I hummed in the hotel bed, lullabying myself to sleep.

. . .

With my three musical projects before that night at Madison Square Garden, I had racked up four-hundred-thousand miles in Ford E350 vans; slept in countless dingy, cheap motel rooms with multiple bandmates crammed into each one; and schlepped my equipment up narrow venue stairwells and through vomit-soaked alleys. Touring with Vampire Weekend, however, was a glimpse into the elite comforts of the music world's stratosphere.

On an overnight flight to Europe, I had fallen asleep in a lie-flat seat, wearing the tie-dye pajamas that our guitar player, Brian, had made for me for my birthday. As we were beginning the descent into Edinburgh the next morning, I was awakened by the gentle tap of a flight attendant who asked, "Madam, may I offer you a French press of coffee?" I wondered: *Was I the only person dressed in head-to-toe tie-dye who had ever been called* Madam?

In a series of surreal backstage encounters, I had brushed shoulders with my idols. I watched the Cure from the side-stage at Glastonbury Festival, passed Emmylou Harris in a hotel hallway, stood next to Nick Cave and his wife in a festival catering line, and caught a glimpse of Robert Plant sipping tea in our hotel lobby in England. Anytime I saw one of these musical gods, I tried to witness them without being noticed, as though I were watching an endangered species in the wild.

When we played the 2018 Fuji Rock Festival in Japan, Bob Dylan was technically the headliner but he didn't want to take the stage after 10 p.m. that night, so he asked to play *before* us. As he exited the stage, our stage tech, Josh, nudged me and said, "That opening act sure knows how to write a banger. I think he's going places."

In Tokyo, the band went out for omakase dinners, enjoying mind-blowing dishes of bluefin toro that tasted like the deep sea, uni that melted like butter in my mouth, Wagyu steak skewers torch-seared to perfection, and ice cream in flavors of miso, lavender, black sesame, and matcha. We sipped sake at a private speakeasy where guests were invited to drink in silence to fully experience each flavor. The host offered poetic descriptions for each glass: "This one tastes like mist after rain," he said. "This one tastes like a cloud from heaven."

In a private karaoke room, we one-upped each other with unexpected songs. Our lead singer, Ezra, blasted through "Chop Suey!" by System of a Down. Our bassist, Chris Baio, crooned "Something Just Like This" by Coldplay and the Chainsmokers. Danielle Haim, who had joined us for that tour, performed "I Don't Want to Wait" by Paula Cole before I launched into "Semi-Charmed Life" by Third Eye Blind. The night ended with a rip-roaring group sing-along of "Mr. Brightside" by The Killers.

Around my Vampire Weekend bandmates, I played up my kid-sister energy, the tomboy aspect of my personality that I'd cultivated growing up with my older brother, surrounded by his friends. At rehearsals and shows, I dressed in men's cargo pants and button-down shirts, wove my long hair into tight braids. But alone in my hotel rooms, I wore lace nightgowns and let my hair down in billowing waves. The boys teased me with affection, as they would a little sister. When we landed in Australia in 2018, I didn't know that airport customs had strict rules against foreign produce. I tried to breeze through security with some olive pits and a few uneaten tomatoes in the container of a salad I'd eaten in transit. After a sniffer dog found the leftovers, the customs officer threatened me with a $2,000 fine. I got off with a warning, but for the rest of the tour, the guys called me "the Salad Bandit."

Touring meant sidelining other parts of myself. No matter what I was feeling backstage, I put on an upbeat persona to perform. When we were due to play Anaheim, I learned that my close friend and musical collaborator Richard Swift was dying at a hospital in Washington. Mutual friends asked me to record a goodbye video that could be played for him during his final days. In the parking lot of the venue, I tried to cram my gratitude for years of his friendship, humor, and creative inspiration into a few minutes of video, then wiped away my tears and stepped onstage. Another time I was laid out backstage with debilitating period cramps, before taking the stage and dancing for a two-and-a-half-hour set, the equivalent of jogging four miles according to my fitness tracker. My body and heart begged me for rest and for tenderness, but the adrenaline of each show kept me pushing my limits.

Exhausted backstage, I often found myself in a state of distraction, scrolling on my phone, disconnected from myself. I spent hours on social media researching a crush who, back in the real world, hadn't texted me back. I tallied up the tour dates and record reviews of other female indie artists my age in some kind of indie-rock keeping-up-with-the-Joneses. I multitasked so often that I rarely felt fully present in a moment. Even when I was on the phone with someone I loved, I was often picking out show clothes or playing scales on my keyboard with the volume turned down.

The crushing exhaustion felt worth it because I was building a nest egg to cover the next year's living expenses and a budget to record my next solo album. I collected dozens of voice memos with some of the biggest melodies I'd ever written, but the lyrics wouldn't come. Between the original songs and covers, Vampire Weekend had a ninety-six-song catalog, and we played a different set every night. Keeping all those songs fresh in my mind required such musical focus that I didn't have much mental space left over for my own songs.

I tried to rebuild my attention span and my connection to myself by doing an hour-long meditation practice each day for a hundred days in a row. Either I'd do it on the tour bus, or I'd sneak up to the highest seats of a theater and meditate in the back row before sound check. During one meditation practice, the venue blasted Poison and Mötley Crüe and I used the sonic assault as a challenge to seek equanimity.

Beneath the euphoria of our sold-out shows and the revelry of our backstage family life, my body sent quiet signals of distress. Flying all over the world and sleeping in different rooms each night was gnawing away at my nervous system. My body was not prepared for the global upheavals I was about to experience.

On New Year's Day 2020, I was trapped in my Sydney hotel room because smoke had blanketed the city: our Australia tour coincided with the worst wildfire season in the country's history. The New Year's Eve festival had been canceled, and tens of thousands of people in high-risk areas had to be evacuated, many on boats out to sea. "Please tell me you're all right," my mom texted. "All I see on the news are burning koalas."

I watched people on the street below walk with T-shirts or scarves shielding their faces. I spent the entire day in bed reading about the climate crisis, my heart sinking with the combination of the information in my hand and the immediate devastation outside my window. On the pad of hotel stationery, I doodled mock-ups for personalized solar-powered temperature-controlled bodysuits.

My body felt like a fuse box on the verge of overload. When we traveled to cleaner air in Melbourne, I was warming up my voice when I noticed a faint flickering of weakness in the upper registers. It felt like cobwebs had formed in the attic of my voice—this tiny quivering sensation, as if I had slightly less control. I blamed the quiver on smoke irritation and jet lag. When I had toured as an opening act for the Zombies in 2014, the singer Colin Blunstone had told me that he adds a minute to his vocal warm-up for every year that he ages. My instinct was to push through and add extra warm-up time. In sixteen years of touring, I'd never lost my voice or canceled a show. I dismissed the idea that something could be seriously wrong.

On our westward journey back to California, we crossed nineteen time zones, stretching the day into a forty-three-hour travel marathon. I pushed through the exhaustion. I was plagued by the irrational fear that someone else was writing the exact same songs as I was, waiting to take my place in the music world. I wanted to launch my solo record the moment the Vampire Weekend album cycle ended, riding the wave of being the band's first female member.

When I arrived home from that tour in 2020, I was determined to spend more time working on my own projects. I began what I secretly referred to as "Stardom Bootcamp," a routine in which every hour of the day was devoted to a different aspect of my musical life. From 8 to 11 a.m., songwriting at the piano; 11 a.m. to 1 p.m., vocal training; 1 to 3 p.m., exercise. Even when I was exhausted, I hiked five to ten miles and went to hot yoga, always in pursuit of a body *just* a bit stronger and sleeker than mine.

In the afternoons and evenings, I often recorded demos, saw friends, or watched music documentaries. In between, I read and meditated and hiked my favorite trails. I didn't want to devote too much time to the quieter aspects of my personality because I didn't feel that they would help me achieve the dream I was envisioning.

After a monthlong break at home in LA, I was back on the road. In March 2020, we headed to play the Okeechobee Music and Arts Festival in Florida. Every other major festival that weekend had been canceled because of the spreading coronavirus, but management deemed this one to be safe because it was a small, local festival that didn't attract many international travelers. We flew to Miami, where a tour bus picked us up. On the four-hour drive to the festival grounds, the newsreel rolled across the bus's television screen:

**ITALY LOCKS DOWN THE COUNTRY'S
NORTH OVER CORONAVIRUS.
NURSING HOMES MOST VULNERABLE
TO CORONAVIRUS.
"JUST STAY CALM. IT WILL GO
AWAY," SAYS US PRESIDENT.**

We huddled together before the TV, and our bass player, Chris Baio, said, "It's been an honor playing with you all. Let's have a great last show." He didn't *really* believe we'd cancel the next ten months' worth of shows, did he? We were supposed to headline festivals in South America with the Strokes starting in two weeks, a tour I'd been looking forward to for months. This virus wouldn't keep me from touring with the Strokes, would it? We were still going to South America, weren't we?

Days after we returned from Okeechobee, I walked my usual neighborhood loop up to Moon Canyon. One moment the sidewalk stretched out in a straight line ahead, and the next, it began spinning in my field of vision like the second hand of a clock. Disoriented, I fell to my hands and knees on the sidewalk, clinging to the ground as the world spun around me. When I tried to stand up, I lost my balance and fell back down, my hands and knees scraping against the concrete.

Cloudy streaks of palm leaves circled above me. The magenta bougainvillea was suddenly so bright that it made me wince. A distant siren blared and the sound felt like a screwdriver piercing my ears. I steadied myself against a palm tree to stand up, then lurched toward a mailbox, braced myself against it, and reached for a bright red car hood, radiant with heat. I found my neighbor's wire fence, and one hand at a time, I steadied myself back to my own yard. My vision was so blurry that it took a few tries to slide my key in the front door lock, and my heartbeat was so loud in my ears that it drowned out the rickety window air conditioner and the sound of my neighbor's Ranchera music.

From bed, I called my best childhood friend, Samantha, who now lived a few miles away. "Something is wrong," I said.

"With the entire world, you mean?" Samantha asked.

The World Health Organization had just declared a global pandemic, the NBA had canceled its season, restaurants and shops had been forced to close their doors, and California had issued a "Safer at Home" order, quite a euphemism for a state-sanctioned lockdown.

"My vision went blurry . . . everything started spinning . . . there's this piercing pain in my temples," I said.

She gave me the words. *Vertigo. Migraine. Migraine aura.* She offered to come over, but I didn't want her to break the quarantine orders.

"I'll keep my phone on tonight," she said. "I can be there in ten minutes anytime you call."

Within hours, violent, shaking chills overtook my body and my throat felt like I'd swallowed a pincushion. As my fever rose, I felt so weak that my water glass seemed to weigh twenty pounds. The next day, I called a family friend who was a doctor and told him I'd just played in Florida, now known to be a COVID hot spot. He suggested that I ride it out at home with liquids and rest.

By the third day, my body was an unlivable planet, too hot for a human to survive and with gravity so powerful that I couldn't stand up. My temperature was 103. My shaking chills were so intense that even as I clutched a heating pad to my body and blasted my space heater, I couldn't get warm.

I shifted in and out of consciousness, and by nightfall, I considered calling Samantha to ask her to take me to the emergency room. But my phone was on a desk by the door, impossibly far away. I caught my reflection in the mirror across the room and my skin was tissue paper white. I felt transparent.

In the middle of the night, I fell into a deep sleep and dreamed that a ghostly figure floated in through the front door. This ashen specter was shaped like the flame of a candle, almost like the grim reaper, but levitating and with fluttering dark edges. The figure hovered over my bed, gazing down at me. In that strange state of consciousness, I could feel that I was dreaming but couldn't wake myself up. The specter said, "Take all your Ambien, every pill at once," with a voice that crackled like a burning campfire.

I'd forgotten about the Ambien. I'd taken one, six months ago, to combat jet lag but was so woozy the next day that I had stashed the remaining pills in my desk drawer and never thought of them again. *Wake up!* I begged myself in the dream. *Wake up! Wake up!* A bolt of fear shocked me awake, my heart racing, my body drenched in sweat. The room was dark other than moonlight reflecting a watery glow on the white upright piano. The figure was gone but there was a lingering presence, as if a real person had just been standing there.

Electrified by this jolt of cortisol, I walked to my desk and fumbled through the drawers, pulling out matchbooks and condoms and crumpled-up sticky notes until I found the aluminum tray of Ambien pills. *Just a dream*, I told myself. *The most psychedelic fever dream.* But something about it felt so real that I worried the nightmare figure could return. I dropped the pills into the toilet one by one and flushed them.

Back in bed, I curled my knees up to my chest like a scared child. I clasped my hands together and did the only thing that I could possibly think of: I prayed. I prayed to the God of my childhood, a God I hadn't communicated with in a long, long time. *Please let me live to see the morning. I'll do anything. I'll live for beauty and truth. No more bullshit, I promise. Please, please, let this fever break.* I was apologizing for all the ways I'd been subtly sabotaging my life: squandering my attention in states of distraction, losing sight of my own creativity, causing myself unnecessary suffering by pursuing unavailable people, taking for granted the people and places I loved most, listening absent-heartedly to the people I loved, and not taking the space to tend to and cherish my body.

A void of dark and deep sleep overtook me for almost twelve

hours, and when I opened my eyes, I heard the shockingly loud symphony of birdsong. The world had stopped spinning and I could walk in a straight line without any wobbling. In the kitchen, the chill of ice-cold water traveled down my throat and cooled my lungs. *Are the birds always this loud?* I wondered. I squeezed an overripe lemon into a second glass of water and the flavor was explosive, bitter, sublime.

In a steaming shower, I shampooed the dried sweat from my scalp. Afterward, I slipped on a clean blue silk nightgown and stepped outside to air-dry my hair in the crisp spring morning. I lay on the hammock and gazed up at the sky, hummingbirds and butterflies fluttering in and out of my field of vision. Distant sirens filled the air, but I imagined turning down the volume of those human-made machines and turning up the volume of the birds. The warm wind caressed my legs and ankles.

Earlier that year, I had seen my neighbors carry their new-born baby outside for the first time. I heard the mother say to the baby, "Look, sweetie, see that up there? That is the sky." Can you imagine seeing the sky for the first time? That's how I felt gazing up through the trees in my backyard.

• • •

There are two seasons in Los Angeles—green season and brown season—and spring 2020 was the lushest green season I'd ever seen. The orange-y layer of smog cleared from the horizon: no one was driving to work.

Weeks after my illness, my body still felt fragile. A constant, dull sore throat made it difficult to swallow, and I had to *gulp* with extra effort. I was winded walking my usual gentle neighborhood hills, and a sandpapery cough appeared whenever I spoke more than a few sentences in a row.

My vocal coach, Allie Martin, invited me to try a lesson online, and though I bristled against shoehorning my real-life experiences onto the screen, it gave me hope to put something on my empty calendar. Monday. Two p.m. A vocal lesson. I'd been taking lessons with Allie since December 2019, in preparation for making a vocally demanding album. Before lockdown, she taught lessons out of her house in West Hollywood, a sanctuary of sobriety, with crystals and copies of the Alcoholics Anonymous Big Book scattered around.

"How are you, Allie?" I asked, as her smiling face appeared on the Zoom screen.

"Still sober!" she said, flexing her bicep like Popeye. She demonstrated a vocal exercise using a *gee-gee-gee-gee* sound up and down the octave. When I sang it back to her, my voice caught in my throat and I couldn't access the highest pitches.

"That's weird," I said. She looked as perplexed as I felt. It was a more visceral and intense version of the gentle flickering I'd felt in my voice in Australia.

I tried again with more breath and effort, but the syllables fell apart in my mouth. The sound in my upper register was like the *Jurassic Park* raptor, all air and screech, no tone.

"It feels like there's a knot in my throat, and when I try to sing high up, the knot gets tighter," I said.

She offered a softer consonant. *Mum-mum-mum-mum.* I

sang it back and the same thing happened. The whole top of my range was gone. Where was my voice? What on earth was happening? She suggested I go see Dr. Peter D. Ashford, a Beverly Hills ENT, if the issue didn't resolve in a few weeks. "For now, let's call it," she said. "Rest up. Drink water. We'll regroup soon."

The issue didn't resolve, and the "few weeks" turned into months because Dr. Ashford's office didn't reopen until July. I made an appointment. His walls were lined with platinum records by the kinds of artists you hear playing at the grocery store. He asked me who I sang with and when I said Vampire Weekend, he said, "Sounds spooky."

Dr. Ashford performed a laryngoscopy, sending a thin camera up my nose and all the way through the nasal passages till it curved down over the vocal cords. I *eeee*-d and *aaaah*-d as instructed.

Watching the video replay, I was shocked to discover that vocal cords look eerily like a tiny singing vagina. Dr. Ashford pointed out a little patch of vocal cord that looked slightly red. He diagnosed me with acid reflux. He prescribed over-the-counter antacids and told me to quit all the foods that make life worth living—coffee, hot sauce, wine, garlic, onions, chocolate, sparkling water.

I wanted to believe Dr. Ashford was right, not only because I had paid $1,200—nearly a month's rent—for the appointment, but also because if the diagnosis was correct, my voice would return in a few weeks. I quit coffee cold turkey and drank sad cups of decaffeinated green tea that tasted like fresh-cut grass.

I ate oatmeal and rice cakes and drank aloe vera juice. I took over-the-counter antacids. I was, not to brag, a perfect patient.

While I waited for the acid reflux to subside, I had nowhere to be and nothing to do. From the whirlwind of touring to sudden lockdown, it was as though I'd gone from driving one hundred miles per hour on the highway to five miles per hour on a dirt road. In an act of great generosity, the Vampire Weekend team offered to pay all band members for the tours that had been canceled. For the first time in my life, I was being paid to *not* work. I had all the time and space I craved, but the early days of the pandemic were so disorienting and unsettling that my mind and body refused to rest. I followed the sunlight around the house like a cat. In the afternoons, I sunbathed in a patch of it in the backyard. Through the chain-link fence, I watched my four-year-old neighbor, Zora, playing next door.

"If I run really fast, I can disappear," she told me one day. "Watch me!" Zora sprinted across the yard and I played along.

"Where did Zora go? Oh, no! We lost Zora!" I yelled. "Can you teach me how to disappear, too?"

"Nuh-uh," she said, shaking her head. "You have to be magic to do it," and she ran off.

To my surprise, her comment actually stung. As a little kid, I had felt the livingness of every plant and rock and animal around me. I spent hours at the creek behind our house examining black frogs small enough to sit on the pad of my pinkie finger. When I held the frogs, I swore I could hear their voices. They laughed with me, they asked about my day, they said *ouch* when they didn't want to be held anymore. I wrote hundreds of songs and stories in made-up languages. And when I did that, I *did* disappear. I, Greta, got out of the way, so that the world could rush in and I could experience it with so much immediacy that I didn't know where I ended and where it began. But lately, when I wrote, it felt like there was a wall between me and the world. I feared Zora was right: I had outgrown the magic.

They call it *playing music* but I seemed to have forgotten the *play* part. I longed to remember how to create the way children do, without fear or hesitation or questions like *Will other people like this? What does this say about me? Is this better than the music that so-and-so just released?*

I'd always thought about my voice as having two sides: the side that sang *out*—to audiences, to my bandmates, to the world beyond me—and the side that sang *in*—accessing and then revealing the contents of my subconscious mind. Without my voice, I felt as though I couldn't access or understand the tangled mess of stress and emotion in my inner world.

Unable to sing outright, I tried to write songs by whistling melodies, but I found it impossible to write lyrics without being able to physically bring them into being. My singing voice was part of my songwriting process, and how I deciphered my emotions. I remember when the line "You're the hurricane I'll never outrun" came out of my mouth during a group songwriting session when I was nineteen. I had written it using my usual Fumble Mumble Method, singing gibberish phrases over and over until words eventually came. "La la la da da dum" turned into "I want an omelet." Eventually, I landed on "You, you're a hurricane . . ."

Once the word *hurricane* was there, a phrase came into being: "the hurricane I'll never outrun." Only after the song was finished did I realize that it referred to my mother's inability to move on after my parents' divorce. I saw how my mother had guarded her heart like a city that had been ravaged by a storm, fearful of another devastation. I hadn't consciously pinpointed that feeling before writing those lyrics. My songs have always told me the truth long before my conscious mind could.

There were so many stories I'd wanted to tell, but they felt too big to put into song. My heart ached for a deep romantic connection and a shared home, like the partnership I had in my twenties, but I'd spent the recent years starving in scraps-of-love relationships with unavailable people. In 2016, I'd written a breakup album called *Midnight Room*. Now, writing breakup songs made me feel like a caricature of a tortured songwriter, reaching for minor 7 chords at the piano while a single, shining tear streamed down my face.

The last song I'd written had been in February, and it had arrived like a transmission, effortlessly, all in one piece. I found song imagery by closing my eyes and conjuring a mental picture, almost like actively dreaming. An image came from a night on tour years before: Cricket song filled the air as I pulled into a hotel parking lot in Corsicana, Texas, at 3 a.m. I schlepped my suitcase across the asphalt, exhausted, and then felt sad when I closed the hotel door and could no longer hear the crickets. Then, the next image I saw was the face of my friend Richard Swift, his eyes wide and alarmed, as if he'd seen something in

the field that I couldn't see. The images didn't make sense together. I'd never been to Corsicana with Richard, who'd died
two years earlier. The lyrics came:

Corsicana lightning
Made my hair stand on end
Out here with the summer snakes again
The crows are laughing at me
I lost my only friend
Out here with the summer snakes again
In a little while you'll see
I was only pretending
In a little while you'll see
My love is never-ending
In a little while you'll see
I was only pretending
He'll come back and find me
This can't be the end
Out here with the summer snakes again

When I demoed that song in December of 2019, I sang deep
in my vocal range, and it felt strange and haunted, like something Bobbie Gentry would sing. "In a little while you'll see I
was only pretending" felt like it came from Richard's perspective, as if he were saying, *Death is just pretending, I'm not really
gone, no one's ever really gone.* I'd started treating songs more like
dreams, allowing them to unfurl through me without having to
understand what they meant.

But just months later, during that first summer of the pandemic, when I closed my eyes for images, my mind was like a dark screen. On an inspired day, songwriting would feel like dipping my bucket into a well and pulling up a refreshing drink of water, but during that writer's block, I felt like I was trying to coax moisture from a parched, cracked rock bed without any luck.

I was tired of writing sorrowful songs from the shadowed waters of my heart. I wanted to write something joyful, maybe a love song, or an anthem to be played at the end of this collective chaos, a soundtrack for brighter times. But every lyric I tried to write that summer of 2020 felt too small and meaningless compared to the pandemic, the fever pitch of the social justice movement, and the climate crisis.

And without a working voice, it was impossible to translate the stories of my life into song.

I expected my voice to improve, but after a few weeks on Dr. Ashford's regimen, the quiver worsened and my voice buckled when I tried to project. There was still a constant, swollen, dull ache and a lump in my throat that required exaggerated effort to swallow. Whenever my voice did strange things, I recorded audio memos into my phone, hoping it might help Dr. Ashford connect the dots. I called him to ask when I should expect improvement. His response was abrupt. "I can't answer that," he said. "Could take one month. Could take four months. Every case is different."

Before joining Vampire Weekend in 2018, when I had toured the country in vans for fourteen years, my body had been like an unstoppable tank. Despite countless overnight driving shifts, gas-station meals, excessive coffee and NoDoz caffeine pills, hours of lugging equipment, and practically screaming to be heard over loud music, my voice had never faltered. I'd always had a perfect health record and a strong constitution. I'd been pushing and pushing my body without anticipating that it might push back someday. I never considered that my voice, my most reliable tool of expression, could disappear in such a strange and sudden way. Being able to sing seemed as essential to feeling like myself as the sun rising is essential to having a tomorrow.

During those early pandemic months, Los Angeles looked like a ghost town with its shuttered shopwindows and empty streets. I took long, slow walks feeling like a foreigner in the city. And without the ability to sing, I felt like a stranger in my own body.

TWO

SOMEONE WHO
NEEDED TO WRITE
SONGS

FROM THE MOMENT I ENTERED THE WORLD, I WAS EXPECTED TO be the happy one. My mom loved to tell the story of my birth: "You looked up at me and smiled. You were beaming. Overjoyed to be in this world."

My mom kept a journal of my early development and gifted it to me when I turned eighteen. She wrote this about me during my first few weeks: "She was born with a sweet, gentle nature. Rarely crying, easily satisfied with soft words of love or tender touch, all qualities we want to encourage throughout life." Whenever I veered out of that state of serene happiness, my mom wrote in the journal, "This is so unlike her." Like the time I'd dressed up in her clothes, as I often did, and came downstairs wearing a negligee, a bustier, and the tiara from the Miss Teen America pageant of her youth. When she forced me to change out of the ensemble before we went out for dinner, I wailed for an hour.

Our house was in the western suburbs of Chicago on a street called Happy Lane, which was lined with weeping willows, maples, and cottonwoods. My family moved there when my older my brother, Garrett, was born. Eighteen months later, I joined them. Wildflowers erupted in our garden, lightning bugs glimmered in the air, and an ice cream truck meandered down the street on summer nights while we played baseball on the cul-de-sac.

When I was almost two, my mom wrote: "My only concern is her lack of fear. She'll try anything Garrett does. Climbing, jumping, swimming, wrestling." I imitated him in every way; I even tried to pee standing up. I did ballet and karate, and then insisted on joining the baseball team like him. "You mean softball?" my parents asked. "Baseball," I said. "With the boys." My parents petitioned the local baseball league and I joined an all-boys team, where I spent most of my time in right field, watching the weeds grow. I grew comfortable being the only girl playing with the boys. They were a bit older and had more freedom—they climbed bigger trees, watched movies I wasn't allowed to see, and could be wilder, dirtier, sweatier, more bruised and scabbed-up than "cute" little girls like me were expected to be.

Every day I sat under the piano with our yellow dog, Gracie. Music encircled us, as if we were in a cave made of sound. My mom played "Ave Maria," the favorite song of her mom—my grandmother, Muriel—who had recently died of a heart attack at age sixty. "I play it for Grammy M," my mom said. My mom usually radiated an inner sunshine, and people were drawn toward her like sunflowers. But when she played "Ave Maria," she withdrew into a place within herself where I wasn't allowed to go. One day I asked, "How does Grammy M hear the song if she's dead?" At the time, my mom believed in a Catholic afterlife, so she said, "She's listening from heaven right now."

Back then, the meaning of the word *dead* was still fuzzy to me. *Dead* was what happened to the silver minnow I won at the carnival and never took out of the plastic bag. *Dead* was what happened to the black garden snake that slithered in front of my brother's bike before he could brake. This notion—that music could be played by someone who was here and heard by someone who was not—exploded like a white firework in my mind.

I already believed that, like in Disney movies, songs were like spells, able to transform the world. In *The Little Mermaid*, Ariel's "Part of Your World" transformed her wish of walking on the land into reality. When my mom told me that my grandmother could hear this song in heaven, music became even more powerful. I climbed up onto the piano bench and pressed the bass notes while she played. I needed to learn this magical language.

Soon, my mom enrolled me in preschool music classes, where I wrote musical notation before I'd learned the alphabet. I scribbled tiny, circular notes into melodies between the staves and begged my mother to play what I'd written. She embellished the melodies as she performed them.

"I wrote that?" I asked, my eyes widening.

"Yes, you did," she said, labeling it Greta's Opus No. 1.

Many hours a day, she hammered away at her typewriter, arcs of paper hanging off the edge of it like synchronized swimmers frozen mid-dive. *Rat-a-tat-tat. Rat-a-tat-tat.* At night, after she washed her face, she smelled like salty ocean air and flowers after rain. While we snuggled in, the warm glow of the TV illuminated her face as she watched *The Mary Tyler Moore Show.* "I used to do that," she once said, pointing to Mary on the screen. "Before I was your mommy, I worked in television like her."

Garrett and I insisted that she write us a fresh bedtime story every night, but they always had to start the same way: *Captain Hook is sailing his pirate ship down the creek and he has almost reached our house . . .*

My dad was a lawyer who was away much of the time working a job I never quite understood. A waterfall of ties hung in his closet, and I used to stand in the midst of them all, pretending I was in a swirling car wash. He spent weeks at a time in foreign countries, and when my mom played us his voicemails from the machine, I used to talk back to the little black box, not understanding that he wasn't actually there. My dad loved music, and when he was home on the weekends, he would ride the exercise bike in the basement in the mornings and sing along at high volume, tone-deaf, to his favorite songs. In the evenings, I danced with him, my feet on his feet, my tiny hand in his giant hand. He had dark eyes, a prominent nose, and a kind, off-center smile. Everyone said I didn't look like him at all.

Stepping through the carved oak and stained glass doors of Immaculate Conception grade school, I was shocked to discover that my creativity, which was always encouraged at home, became a one-way ticket to hell. At Immaculate Conception, Catholic nuns taught us that we were all born sinners and we had to pray if we wanted to go to heaven. I used to imagine that heaven was an invisible celestial cloud palace floating above the shopping mall and hell was an invisible lake of fire underneath the local McDonald's.

My mom wove my sun-bleached hair into elaborate French braids like Gretl, the youngest Von Trapp child in *The Sound of Music*. "Do you sing like Gretl?" people often asked when I introduced myself, but I was shy with my voice. When my classmates sang church hymns during Friday mass, I just whispered. My voice felt too personal to share. Alone, though, I sang constantly. To the moon, to the flowers, to my dog. The night I learned to ride my bike without training wheels, I spun hundreds of circles around the cul-de-sac while the sky turned peachy-gold and dandelion dust floated in the air. I wrote melodies in a secret language for hours.

When I was nine, I wrote a story about two friends who travel to hell, that fiery furnace beneath McDonald's, searching for a time-traveling manual. When I read it out loud, my classmates were a rapt audience—that is, until the teacher gasped and silenced me mid-sentence. The smell of chalk dust and funeral incense burned my nostrils, and I watched the faces of my classmates change one by one like a jury being convinced of my guilt. In the thick silence, my face burned hot with shame.

In her office, the principal reprimanded me. "Hell is not a joke, Greta."

"I wasn't telling a joke," I said. "I was telling a *story*." My body broke out in a stress rash beneath my scratchy, starched uniform.

"Be a good girl," she commanded. "Stop telling stories about hell."

At piano lessons, I also got in trouble—for remixing Beethoven. I scanned my sheet music and grabbed a few chords, then created a repeating pattern and added my little lines of poetry over them.

"Play Beethoven the way Beethoven wrote it," my teacher said. She told me there was no point in writing my own songs because the only way to earn a living in music was to become a teacher like her.

In our basement, I was free: My dad's Wurlitzer jukebox was a portal to a secret world. My fingers would reach up, pressing buttons on the glowing machine, and the speakers would fill with a warm, crackling sound. The songs spoke of the ecstasy of love, the agony of heartbreak, the longing for freedom, the despair of oppression. They expressed wilder emotions than anything I'd ever seen in real life.

When I get that feeling, I want sexual healing, sang Marvin Gaye.

At age six, that song made me blush, though I couldn't explain what sexual healing was.

Billie Jean is not my lover, sang Michael Jackson, as he claimed that a child didn't belong to him.

At age seven, I wondered what a lover had to do with a son.

Hello darkness, my old friend, sang Simon and Garfunkel.

At age eight, I wondered how darkness could be a friend, considering how scary it was.

They paved paradise and put up a parking lot, sang Joni Mitchell.

At age nine, it seemed preposterous that anyone would trade palm trees for asphalt.

The songs were like keys opening doors within me that I never even knew *existed*. Many years later, I would learn that the word *stanza* comes from the Italian word for *room*. That's what it felt like: with every verse, I was entering a new room, a new world.

At school, my friends were all named after saints. I forced them to play "band" with me on the playground, jamming on imaginary instruments and singing backup vocals. My dedication to the playground band was so unwavering that I once sought my mom's advice on a crucial decision: One of our vocalists always sang off-key after getting her braces tightened. Did I need to "fire" her or just postpone practices to fall on non-orthodontic days? Mom said she should stay.

Then, at age ten, I found a copy of my mom's photographic Kama Sutra book, in which nude models demonstrated sexual poses. The songs on the jukebox were suddenly making sense. I took the book to school, and like a detective reaching the climactic *a-ha* moment of solving a crime, I exclaimed to my bandmates, "I think I understand how babies are made!"

When my friends told their parents that I had taught them what sex was, I was disinvited from all the upcoming slumber parties and forbidden from entering their homes. The playground band broke up. My mom's best friend joked that there was only one solution: "Your family is going to have to move."

Instead, I transferred to a new school that emphasized the arts. We tapped maple trees to make syrup, made short films on 16mm cameras, and learned how to swing dance. My new friends were Jewish and Muslim and Hindu, and I loved the aromatic food at their houses and the colorful gods of Eastern theology. Best of all, there were no more scratchy uniforms, and no one told me I was going to hell anymore.

After school, my mom often asked, "How are your PIES?" This was her acronym meaning that she wanted to hear about the Physical, Intellectual, Emotional, and Spiritual aspects of my life. Though I often shrugged my way through her line of questioning, my PIES had all improved since entering a school for the arts.

Soon after I transferred, an even bolder mischief-maker replaced me at Immaculate Conception—Eileen. When she blazed into that school with whoopee cushions in her pocket and a hot pink training bra under her uniform shirt, my former classmates told us that we needed to meet. When Eileen and I were introduced at a local fair, we were like two puzzle pieces clicking into place. We looked so much alike that we dressed as twins on Halloween.

A few months later, we wandered Nordstrom's while my mom ran an errand. Eileen pulled a $4,500 dress off the rack and tried it on in the dressing room. The clerk scolded her, saying, "Don't you understand? That's a Chanel!" Eileen immediately went into character. "Don't *you* understand? I am Zsa Zsa Gabor and I need to look beautiful for my special occasion!" Eileen and I became so close that our parents' most effective punishment was to separate us for a weekend.

• • •

In 1999, when I was eleven, I thought Y2K would be the end of the world. At least that's what the news made it seem like, that the coming turn of the millennium would cause a fatal disruption in computer technology. I lay awake late at night imagining that, on New Year's Eve, airplanes would drop out of the sky, nuclear bombs would be detonated, bank records would be erased, and the world as we knew it would descend into chaos. Amid my apocalypse anxieties, I never expected a more intimate and imminent collapse: my family as I knew it would come to an end.

In the summer of 1999, my mom had taken me and my brother to Santa Fe, New Mexico, for a family vacation. We'd been going to Santa Fe every summer for my dad's law conferences, and my parents loved it so much that they bought an adobe house for their eventual retirement. My dad had told us that he needed to stay behind for work, so he came a few days later. When he arrived, he and my mom went for a walk, and when they returned, my mom's face was pale and expressionless, as though the wind had been knocked out of her.

"We both love you very much," my dad told me and my brother. I sensed it was the beginning of a Bad News Sandwich—that was his technique of "sandwiching" bad news between two pieces of good news. "But we have decided to separate," he said, presenting it as a unified decision. My mom was wearing sunglasses, even though we were inside. Behind them, slow tears rolled down her face.

"I spent the last few days moving into a loft apartment downtown," my dad said. "Two homes means twice the birthday gifts. You can celebrate Hanukkah with me and Christmas with your mom." My mom stayed silent and her hand trembled as she reached for her water glass.

The strangest part was that my parents had seemed so *happy*. They sang along to the radio when we went out for ice cream on summer nights. I remember taking baths while my mom trimmed hair from the back of my dad's neck or while they brushed their teeth side by side, always touching, always tender. On weekend evenings, they often lay opposite each other on the couch rubbing each other's feet. (In adulthood, I call this position "the Hiker's 69.")

In the few years before they split, my mom had become interested in holistic health, and I sensed my dad thought it was cuckoo. Iridologists looked at pictures of our eyes. Acupuncturists treated our headaches. When she read that it was healthier to sleep on a north/south axis, she suggested that we all sleep sideways in our beds. Still, their happiness had felt as real and solid as our house. Was all that affection a charade, or could love as true as theirs actually vanish overnight?

I remembered one fight, years earlier, when my mom whisper-yelled behind their bedroom door after my dad returned from a business trip in China bearing bags of gifts for us.

"You can't just waltz in here like some Jewish Santa Claus! When you bring gifts back from trips, it makes the kids excited for you to go away," she said. My mom showed him a picture my brother had made in art class—he'd been assigned to draw a family portrait, and it included only the three of us, minus my dad, since he was gone so often. My mom said, "What the children need is your *presence*, not your presents."

"How do you think we pay for all this, Anne?" my father said. "This life? This house?"

"We don't need all this," my mom said. "What we need is you."

That night in Santa Fe, after my parents told us they were splitting, my mom and I slept on the roof to watch a meteor shower. Coyotes howled in the distance and a rabbit's high-pitched cry pierced the air. The more she assured me that everything would be okay, the more it sounded like she was trying to convince herself of that. "I will love you so much that you won't even miss Dad," I said.

Our family drove two twelve-hour days from New Mexico back to Chicago. With my headphones blasting music to drown out the conversation, they looked like a normal couple in the front seats, but when we returned to Illinois, my dad hugged and kissed us goodbye and went to sleep at his apartment. Our house looked like we'd been robbed—empty squares on the walls where my father's paintings had hung, a vacant spot in the garage where his car had been, a bare half of their closet.

Inspired by *Harriet the Spy*, I eavesdropped on everyone, copying my observations into a spiral notebook. I used Harriet's technique of holding the phone button down while lifting the receiver, then gently easing the button up. In the days after my dad left, my mom spent hours on the phone with her friend Candy.

"He's leaving me for a *baby* woman?" my mom said. "She's almost half my age." My mom's voice was raw and trembling.

"He's not going to build a life with her," Candy said. "It'll blow over. It's a midlife crisis."

The "other woman" was a young associate at his law firm who admired his unwavering dedication to his craft, a direct counterpoint to my mother, who longed for the time stolen by his work. My mom told Candy that she had found the woman's address and mailed her one of our Christmas cards with the message *THIS IS THE FAMILY YOU DESTROYED!* scrawled in permanent marker. I was terrified by the sound of my mother's voice. She sounded scornful, almost evil—until her voice softened into a whimper. "How could he leave us?" she said, breaking into sobs.

An hour later, my mom emerged from her bedroom performing an eerie charade of her usual upbeat self. "Who wants buckwheat pancakes?" she asked, her voice rising at the end like a radio jingle.

I was so sensitive to the moods and emotions of those around me that I held her heartbreak in my own chest, her grief in my belly. I had no boundaries between my mother and myself. I began looking at myself in the mirror wondering what was wrong with me, why I wasn't good enough. *How could he leave us?*

Months later, my parents reunited with new vows of love, then separated again. After that, my mom went to the emergency room thinking she was having a heart attack. She returned with a prescription for Valium and slept for twenty hours, then filed for divorce. Weeks later, they reunited yet again, and she rescinded the divorce. Soon there was a fight during which my mom threw almost all the dishes from the cabinet on the floor, shattering them one by one until our kitchen looked like a sea of broken china. My dad swept up the broken pieces.

She started primal screaming in the basement at odd hours. She stabbed pillows in the yard, leaving tiny cotton snowdrifts to float across the chive-green summer lawn. She glued cutout magazine photos of Brad Pitt over my dad's face in framed family photos and said to friends, "He's being *something* that rhymes with PITT-head."

Growing up, I'd overheard stories about my maternal great-grandmother Harriet, whom I naturally wanted to know more about since she shared a name with Harriet the Spy. My great-grandmother had returned home one day to discover that her husband was cheating on her and supposedly "lost her mind" afterward. I imagine Harriet was likely experiencing valid rage and grief, but those were the days when women were locked up for *hysteria*. She was institutionalized at a sanitarium, and though little is known about her stay in the hospital, family lore says that she returned home nearly catatonic. She was a distant, cold mother to Muriel, my grandmother, who grew up to become an alcoholic. I wish I knew more about Harriet's life and desires, but unfortunately her shape on our family tree was reduced to a shadowy silhouette and only a few plot points. My mom was the center of my universe, and I worried that this heartbreak could overtake her as it had my great-grandmother.

When my parents reunited a third time, I considered my dad an interloper. As the new millennium came upon us, we spent New Year's Eve as a family in Santa Fe. No planes fell out of the sky, no nuclear bombs went off, no computers exploded. But soon in the new year, my parents took a trip to England and the diamond fell out of my mom's wedding ring on the plane, never to be found. When they returned from the trip, my dad filed for divorce. This time it stuck.

That first year after the divorce, my dad was more physically present than ever before, coming out to the suburbs to take me to dinner and bringing bouquets of flowers to my dance recitals. Mentally, though, he seemed absent, asking the same questions over and over. I wondered whether he had too many cases in his head to remember details about my life. I gave the same answers over and over without acknowledging that we were re-peating ourselves. He cared about my grades so I pretended to care about my grades. He cared about sports so I pretended to care about sports.

When the divorce was final, my mom embarked on a mas-sive home clean-out. The first thing she donated was their bed. She rented a giant dumpster and told me and Garrett to dis-card anything that no longer made us happy. One night she mentioned that she'd thrown out all her journals. "All that pain . . . gone, gone, gone!" she said.

A writer throwing away her journals seemed like a mistake. After she fell asleep, I climbed into the dumpster and dug through the gigantic pile of discarded items with a flashlight. I found five notebooks with large gaps of time between them.

In my room, I thumbed through the journals and found a passage from when she was pregnant with me. In tilted, angry chicken-scratch, she had written: "I feel there is a critical destructive force within me, one that can destroy anyone and anything in its path. Maybe my sweet husband and son would be better off without me and my anger." Who was this woman? Before the recent emotional eruptions caused by the breakup, my mom had always been high-spirited, optimistic, relentlessly creative, sunny-side up. She made siren sounds when we passed blooming gardens, saying, "*WEEEEOOOOO WEEEOOOO* Beauty Patrol!" She called fruit "earth candy." She did yoga sun salutations and spoke self-love affirmations. But this woman on the page once believed she had a critical, destructive force within her. Was my mom's positive outward persona a mask, or was it real? Pangs of guilt pulsed through me and I buried the journals under clothes in my closet and vowed never to read them again without her permission.

To numb the pain I was feeling, I ate and ate, sneaking ice cream from the freezer and smearing bagels with peanut butter and honey. Soon, *you are what you eat* came true on my body: by summer, my waistline looked like a large, round plain bagel.

My Walkman became my most reliable friend. Songs mirrored my inner world experiences in ways my friends couldn't. When songwriters and singers articulated the hazy, aching emotions that were whirling within me, the songs drew those emotions to the surface so I could experience and then release them.

I loved any song that felt like a sugar rush. The glittery pop of the Spice Girls, TLC, NSYNC, and Ace of Base made me dance in the basement for hours. The warm, autumnal drawls of Faith Hill and Alan Jackson made me imagine cinematic kisses in the rain. The adrenaline-rushing raps of Eminem and Dr. Dre made me feel like I could lift a pickup truck with my bare hands. From my *Now! 11* compilation CD, Lenny Kravitz sang, "I wanna get away, I wanna fly away," and I gazed up at the big open sky from a lawn chair thinking, *You and me both, Lenny, you and me both.*

In the early 2000s, my mom read Deepak Chopra's book *Ageless Body, Timeless Mind*, which suggested identifying with a chosen age rather than a biological one. Afterward, she crossed out her date of birth on a few IDs, and began referring to herself as "ageless and timeless." On her birthday each year, when we asked how old she was, she'd say, "I have no idea. Happy ageless and timeless day to me!"

My dad's relationship with the young associate imploded, and soon he met Shelley, a real estate agent from Miami who loved art and design, had impeccable style, had two grown children, was his age, and was even more organized than he was. Shelley began spending time in Chicago, building a relationship that would eventually become a marriage.

Because I was gaining weight, responding to all my mom's daily PIES inquiries with annoyed shrugs, biting my nails till they bled, and barely talking to my dad when he came over for dinner, my parents sent me to their counselor, Dr. Avery. I hated his caterpillar eyebrows, square gray teeth, and the way he spoke to me in a sing-song voice for children.

Far too many sessions went like this:

Dr. Avery: Are you angry with your father for leaving?
Me: Why should I tell *you* anything?

What I felt was the opposite of anger: a wall of ice was forming around me, a glacial quiet, the numbness of unspoken hurt.

In our Irish Catholic suburbs, divorce was rare and considered blasphemous. Eileen, whose own parents had split, was my only friend who understood. While my parents' divorce had made me want to retreat, to shut myself off from romantic love, hers seemed to turn her into a love monster. Every social move she made was fueled by a desire for connection with boys.

In sixth grade, she had the biggest boobs in her class and was hypersexualized by her fellow students because of it. She was light-years ahead of me in romantic experience. When I was twelve and she was thirteen, she dared me into my first kiss by insisting that the boy and I needed to "switch gum" for it to count as Frenching—my Doublemint for his Big Red. That night, I fell asleep kissing my hand, trying to re-create the silky-wet sensation of his tongue.

One summer at the carnival on the Gravitron ride—a circle podium that spun so fast that you couldn't lift your arms or legs because of the centrifugal force of gravity—a boy we knew pulled down her tube top on a dare. He'd had the strength to reach over to do it, but she didn't have the strength to lift her arms to pull it back up, so her exposed breasts flopped side to side. The look on her face was a mix of embarrassment and anger, but when the ride stopped, she pulled her shirt up and I watched her perform a mental calculation. When we gathered with our friends at the exit sign, she laughed with pride, "Guess what? The carny said we can ride as many times as we want for free!"

For five summers, we went to camp together in northern Minnesota. My joy and relief there were so sincere that everyone called me Greta Sunshine. Eileen was my bunkmate and we bathed in the blue-green lake, slept in cabins without running water or electricity, canoed our little hearts out, and treated s'mores as their own food group.

By this time, I'd been writing fragments of melodies and half-formed lyric ideas in my notebooks. I sang my own melodies and added harmonies over my favorite artists' tracks while listening, but I hadn't yet written entire songs front to back.

At the end-of-the-summer campfire, our counselor, Mary Jane, strummed her guitar and sang "The Circle Game" by Joni Mitchell. The song was like an entire movie in four minutes; it taught me everything I needed to know about songwriting.

In the first verse, a little boy catches a dragonfly in a jar and is scared of a thunderstorm. In the chorus, she describes a carousel going around. She says that you can't go back to where you came from, but rather you just "go round and round and round in the circle game." The verses move through time—the boy skates on frozen streams when he's ten, then rolls through town in his car as a teenager. Eventually the singer warns that it won't be long "till you drag your feet to slow the circles down."

The chorus comes around again like a beating heart that pumps life to the rest of the song. Circular images echo throughout: cartwheels, car wheels, the jar containing the dragonfly, the carousel, years spinning by. All these words that sound similar were placed back to back—*painted ponies, captive/carousel.* When she sings "up and down," her melody also moves up and down.

It was the saddest song I'd ever heard.

It felt like we'd just arrived at camp, but somehow two months had gone by and now it was over. I clutched Eileen, both of us in tears, while smoke from the campfire rose up into the humid, mosquito-filled Minnesota air.

Before bed, both of us in our bunks, I said, "We're like the little boy with the dragonflies."

"What are you talking about?" she asked.

"One day, we'll be so old that we'll drag our feet to slow the circles down!"

"Whoa, whoa," she said. "You haven't even been felt up yet! You don't even have your driver's permit yet!" But I feared the quickening of time. Eileen hated feet, so I reached my toes down from the upper bunk and held them close to her face and said,

"You haven't even had your hair brushed with toenails yet!" She squirmed away, laughing, and then we fell asleep.

All summer, I'd crushed on a boy and built an obsessive fantasy that he'd give me an end-of-the-summer kiss goodbye. I made him a friendship bracelet and placed it in an envelope with a note that read *Wear this bracelet to breakfast tomorrow if you like me back!* At breakfast on the final day, his friend hand-delivered the envelope back to me with the bracelet still inside.

When I arrived home, my mom had started writing bluegrass lyrics, inspired by the movie *O Brother, Where Art Thou?* I found a song in the printer called "Rest in Peace," which was about a woman whose only cure for heartbreak insomnia was to imagine that her cheating husband is dead. The chorus refrain said, *Yes, I rest best when you are dead.*

Transitioning back into my homelife, I was carrying an ache too big for my body to handle. My budding breasts were growing and my period now came each month, not like the vampire blood you see in movies, but like red earth in New Mexico. Hormones swirled their chaotic storm through my preteen frame.

I stumbled on a two-track tape deck in the basement, a relic from my mom's television days. I set it up on the keyboard in my room and pressed "record." I tracked one piano part that had a little riff based on a Chopin sonata, then went into a second super-simple three-chord repetition. I played it back, over and over, hoping to create separate verse and chorus sections like "The Circle Game." I sang, my voice hesitant, a shy confession whispered to the room. But then the words, clumsy at first, found their rhythm, tumbling out.

You are the lighthouse
I'm lost at sea . . .
The storm roars and roars
Till I'm shipwrecked
On your shore

Pure teenage poetry, messy and overwrought, but the song came from inside like a light, my inner world expanding outward in circles. I rewound the tape, playing it back over and over, until melodies coalesced. I was practically catching my breath as I wrote the chorus:

What if my broken heart never heals?
What if I never find a love that's real?

My chest felt like a net full of butterflies, all these living, fluttering ideas inside of me. I wrote the lyrics down, crossing out one word and choosing another. The playback was barely audible, the machine warbling and distorted. But it was there: my first full song. I called it "Lost at Sea."

I was so sensitive to the needs and desires of others that, in conversations with people I loved, I chameleoned my voice and presence, performing subtle contortions to fit their moods and expectations. On tape, there was no fawning, no desire to please anyone other than myself. Just a stark, unvarnished, whispered truth, sung from myself to myself.

Years later, I read a *Paris Review* interview with William Maxwell in which he recalled asking Pete Lemay, who had known Willa Cather, what he thought had made Cather a writer. Lemay replied, "Why, what makes anyone a writer—deprivation, of course."

Over time, I noticed that recurring theme in the origin stories of my favorite artists: something crucial was ripped from them, leaving an emptiness. But instead of being consumed by that emptiness, their art flooded into it.

In a 1995 radio interview, Joni Mitchell told the story of being ill with polio at age nine. Formerly an athletic tomboy, she found herself lying in a hospital bed suffering a disease that was often fatal and that threatened to permanently take away her ability to walk. During that time, she said, she developed an acute ability to observe others and also developed an inward gaze. She came to believe that the fertile mind state she cultivated during that time became the source of her eventual outward expressions. Polio had weakened her left hand, so she experimented in her teen years with open guitar tunings, which were easier for her fingers to manage. Those unconventional guitar voicings eventually became her signature style.

Every artist has their own creative Big Bang. Beforehand, the potential for creativity is always there, every spark of possibility condensed into one pinpoint within the heart, but most of us need a catalyst.

My parents' divorce transformed me from someone who *wanted* to write songs into someone who *needed* to write songs. Every day after school, I played piano and sang the way herbalists concoct medicine, listening back to the songs as though dosing myself with the one thing that would heal me. When I couldn't sleep, I wrote my own lullabies. When I ached for unrequited crushes, I turned longing into melodies. Songwriting was a sacred and secret act—a musical diary with an imaginary lock on it. The question of whether my songs were good didn't cross my mind, the same way I wouldn't have questioned whether a life raft was *good* if it was tossed to me while I was drowning.

I could express things in songs that I wasn't brave enough to share in conversation. I could translate the literal experiences of my life into lyrical experiences, veiling the meanings *just* enough to keep them private. Every songwriting session felt like dropping a suitcase that had been too heavy to carry. Afterward, I felt ten feet tall.

• • •

By age thirteen, the sugary melodies of pop were too sweet and I craved the raw energy of punk and grunge. I begged my parents to let me pierce my eyebrow. In a strategic move, they offered that I could do so only if I earned straight A's. I'd wanted to pierce my eyebrow as a way of rebelling against "the System," but now my rebellion was contingent on perfect compliance to its standards. So, instead, I dyed the lower layer of my hair, closest to the nape of my neck, black. I wore my hair down during the day to hide it from my parents, but I tied my hair up in a high ponytail at concerts to reveal my punk energy, the way some birds reveal colorful under-feathers in mating dances.

That year, inspired by the movie *Almost Famous*, I started a music zine with a friend. Interviewing members of dozens of all-male local bands revealed a wild double standard: when women expressed difficult emotions, they were *crazy*, but when men expressed difficult emotions, they were *poetic*.

After I'd wrapped an interview with a local band, they made fun of the lead singer's ex-girlfriend, who'd been so heartbroken after their breakup that she started posting cryptic poems about him on her blog. The guys called her "a handful," "cuckoo," and "high maintenance," and joked that maybe he should weave one of her lyrics into their next single. The next week, when I watched the same band play a local show, he sang about the breakup, and my friends went on and on about how sensitive and mysterious he was.

As I neared age fourteen, Eileen took me to my first few unchaperoned concerts. We saw Weezer and Blink-182 and a handful of other local bands in church basements. I had always attended concerts hoping that the lead singers would notice me, catch my gaze, and see something special in me. Around this time, when I watched male-fronted bands, I began to think that I'd rather be more *like* them than be noticed *by* them.

My bedroom closet had folding mirrored doors. One day, I sang along to a Get Up Kids record into my hairbrush, catching glimpses of myself from various angles, imagining how I would appear to an unseen audience. The dream of becoming a singer began to hover like the sun, too bright to gaze at directly. I orbited around it like a distant planet, each circle bringing me closer to the blazing center of that longing.

I began constructing a vision of my flawless future self: She was talented, beautiful, successful, graceful. She held the crowd in the palm of her hand. She was so beloved and respected that no one would ever break her heart. At fourteen, I decided piano was no longer cool and asked for a gift: a guitar.

Finally, a boy I had a crush on named Tim told my friend Maggie that he liked me, and I told Maggie to tell him I liked him back. Then, boom, I had my first boyfriend. Tim wrote his own songs and played at coffee shops and open mics as a duo with his cousin Ryan. Tim also played drums in a punk band with our friend Bob. Most of the older local guys were in punk and emo bands. Tim taught me how to play my first guitar chords, wrapping his hand around mine to demonstrate C, G, D. During a meal of chicken fingers and French fries at the local Houlihan's, we wrote a contract saying that we would marry each other when we reached age twenty-five. We imagined that, by twenty-five, we'd be *real adults*.

Tim suggested that I sleep with my guitar in bed because he believed that the best songs come to those who keep their instruments close. At my house one day after school, he pointed to the books of poetry on my shelves—by Sylvia Plath, William Blake, Langston Hughes—and prophesied that I'd eventually outshine the male songwriters in our circle. But I guarded my early songs like fragile, newborn birds.

How do you know the gift you are meant to offer the world? Whatever you secretly dream of doing and, simultaneously, are terrified of doing—that's it.

• • •

The room with the best acoustics in my house was the basement bathroom, so that's where the song circle ended up. In 2003, when I was about to turn fifteen, I was hosting a party at my mom's house. Eileen had moved to Connecticut that year, and in her place, I built a community of new friends. After my artsy middle school, I was back in a Catholic private prep high school in the next town, but most of these new friends were public school kids from my neighborhood. Many of them were older than I was and were already playing in local bands.

My friend Bob sat on the closed toilet seat and played a song. He had shaggy ginger hair, blue eyes, and skin that had been pockmarked with teenage acne. He'd been playing in local bands for a few years and desperately wanted to get signed. Bob passed the guitar to our friend Evo, who played a song and passed the guitar to Tim. Tim and I had broken up but we were still close friends. He was the only one who knew I'd been secretly writing songs, so he passed the guitar to me.

My body flooded with fight-or-flight hormones as if I were about to leap out of a plane. It was hard to tell which seemed more terrifying: playing the song or passing the guitar along *without* playing a song. I held the guitar, my hands shaking before I even plucked the strings. I fingerpicked the intro over and over, willing my voice to come through. And then, I dove out of the plane.

Barely louder than a whisper, I sang a version of my song "Echo," which had evolved out of the messy first song, "Lost at Sea," from years earlier.

> *You were the navigator who never could lead*
> *We were lost in the silver sea . . .*

My voice trembled from nerves. The song layered the secret stories of my life and the unmoored feelings I had after my parents split up. Our family was drifting and I didn't know who was navigating.

> *Echo, my voice is an echo*
> *Of places I don't know*
> *And stories I've been told.*

In the bridge, I sang about my extended familial tapestry, my life as a result of all the lives that came before me. These feelings and longings were too nuanced to express to my friends in conversation. They only made sense in songs.

Stress sweat pooled under my arms into the T-shirt beneath my jean jacket. My gaze was zoomed in on the fretboard of the guitar, and in my peripheral vision, I could see Converse sneakers and beer cans covered with droplets of condensation. When I finished, Tim applauded and then everyone else did.

"Holy shit, Greta," he said. "That was beautiful."

"Yeah, for a girl," Bob said.

My friend Samantha, a spunky Irish redhead, said, "Bob, that was a great joke . . . for a guy with turds for brains!"

I passed the guitar along and the circle continued, but a thrilling river of adrenaline kept running through my body. *I did it. I can't believe I did it.*

Listening to the others' songs, I realized that mine was different. The boys wrote earworm melodies with clever one-liners; upbeat, chugging tempos; and catchy riffs. My song was folkier and dreamlike, the lyrics mysterious and cinematic. I sensed that my private musical secrets might actually be worth sharing with others. Once I allowed that inner voice to break through to the world around me, it broadened my sense of identity from being a "regular" kid to being someone who had a special offering: I could express the hidden things that others couldn't say.

Later in the night, Bob apologized. "Your song was better than mine. That's why I was a jerk," he said. "If you ever wanna write together, it would be cool to play music with you." And that was the invitation that would change my life.

THREE

CAN YOU SING IT MORE LIKE THIS?

AFTER THE NIGHT OF THE SONG CIRCLE, BOB AND I WROTE TO-gether after school every day—him at the guitar and me at the piano. I'd usually be in my school uniform—a red and gray plaid skirt, knee-high socks, and button-down uniform shirt with the Benet Academy crest. He'd be in his uniform—ripped jeans, Converse, and a faded Saves the Day T-shirt. We named our project The Hush, inspired by how many times we told my dog, Gracie, to hush her barking while we were writing.

We did free-writes to generate lyrics, each of us filling two to three pages with hyper-vulnerable emotional outpourings and then swapping our notebooks and underlining each other's strongest phrases. My strength was visceral lyrics with images and storytelling, and his was writing big, memorable, sing-along choruses. All my early songs happened lyrics first. During school days, I tucked my song notebook inside whatever textbook I was supposed to be reading and spent class time crossing out rhymes and trying different lyrical lines. Then, when I returned from school, I'd try singing the lyrics at the piano.

In those early days with me and Bob as a two-piece, our writing sessions started to feel like dates. The emotional intimacy of songwriting ignited into a romance. We wrote each other love letters constantly and bought each other new books and vintage T-shirts. Then, while I was away for a summer, he kissed someone else and I broke up with him. I blamed it on the kiss, but the truth was that I wanted to be his bandmate more than his girlfriend.

Soon, we were joined by Darren, a smiley, shy, brown-haired, brown-eyed drummer from two towns over, who started practicing with us in the basement after school. Bob and Darren wanted to be professional musicians, but they were both slogging through community college to earn degrees for jobs they didn't really want. I was entering my sophomore year at college-prep Benet Academy, where we were taught to strive for *excellence* and expected to earn college board scores in the top 1 percent. The school motto was Latin *Ora et labora*, meaning "Pray and Work." I didn't think being a professional musician was actually possible. I wanted to study psychology and music and imagined staying in Chicago to jam with Bob and Darren on the weekends.

My house became the band's central command, the basement transforming into our musical jam zone, with a cheap PA system that gave off shrill flashes of feedback. My mom swore that she loved it when the whole house rumbled, and she stocked the basement kitchen with food from Costco for the boys. Having these musical brothers eased some of the pain of missing my brother, Garrett, who'd left for college in Vermont that year.

Fueled by root beer and mozzarella sticks, and buzzing with teenage hormones, Bob and I channeled our feelings into our songs, as if we were writing a suburban, PG-13 version of Fleetwood Mac's *Rumours*. One crisp fall day during my sophomore year, Darren and Bob tumbled down the basement stairs, flushed and sweaty from wrestling on the trampoline in the yard. I trailed behind, unbuttoning my uniform shirt for that end-of-the-day laziness, revealing a Rilo Kiley shirt peeking out from underneath.

Bob and I had broken up, but he was still trying to win me back. The week earlier, he'd told me, "If you died, I'd want to die, too. That's how much I love you." Days after, we found ourselves stuck in traffic in downtown Chicago. "If you loved me once, then why can't you love me again?" he pleaded.

"I do love you," I said, "but as a friend and bandmate." His face went white, like he was about to throw up.

A friend in Naperville had invited us to play a show in his basement, which would be the first time we played for an audience. At this rehearsal, Bob and I pitched new songs to fill out the set. Bob played his first song idea, "City Traffic Puzzle."

I don't want to love you, he sang, *If love leaves me this cold . . .* It had one of the most memorable and exciting chorus melodies that he'd ever written. And the bridge described the exact moment in the car:

You said no, and I don't think I can take it
This car's caving in
Both so upset
We're lovesick and sick of it.

Darren liked the chorus so much that he couldn't resist playing and dropped in with a rock-and-roll swing beat. *Ting-tinka-ting, tinka-ting, tinka-ting.* I glanced at Bob's hands on the fretboard to see the chords, then played a piano riff over the instrumental section. Once we played through it a few times, we added the song to the *yes* list on the dry-erase board. It was my turn to play, so I strummed a folky guitar rhythm, the kind that sounds like a train rolling down the tracks: *I know that you're an artist*, I whisper-sang, *But you're the hardest one to deal with . . .*

The tension crackled in the room. I didn't want to look at Bob, worried my face would give away the fact that the words were about him. Instead, I looked at Darren, whose mouth flickered into a smile that was both nervous and delighted, as though he knew exactly what the song was about. Bob was territorial around me and inserted himself into any conversation I had with other boys, acting like it was to protect me, when really it felt like it was to possess me.

You painted me in pastels / colors that don't tell of any boldness / That's the way you'd love to see me / So delicate, so weak, so little purpose, I sang.

"What's that about?" Bob asked, sending a sullen stare my way. I panicked and looked around the room. *The Picture of Dorian Gray* was on top of a pile of schoolbooks on the table.

"It's about this book," I said, pulling a connection out of thin air. "This guy, Dorian Gray, has a portrait painted of himself . . . and then the portrait ages while he stays young . . . It's about the artist who painted the portrait." Bob's face relaxed. Darren added a shuffle drumbeat, Bob played a folky guitar riff over it, and we added the song to the *yes* board.

Then, Bob strummed the opening chords to a song called "Momentum" while he stared at his notebook sitting on the floor in front of his feet. *You are the dark ocean bottom*, he sang, his voice a low, longing rumble. *And I am the fast-sinking anchor.* His eyes flickered up to meet my gaze.

Then he belted the angsty chorus: *All we need is a little bit of momentum to break down these walls that we've built around ourselves.* I winced, feeling guilty that I wasn't able to give him what he wanted. Then again, by *not* dating him, I'd inspired his best songs. Darren and I both applauded, and I added it to our dry-erase board of *yes* tunes.

By the end of practice, we had eight songs and we played them back-to-back. Our set flowed the way an eight-course meal might. Something salty, then something sweet. Upbeat, anthemic excitement, then a low-key ballad palate cleanser, followed by some humorous banter to uplift, followed by a call-and-answer song to engage the crowd.

None of our individual voices was particularly extraordinary, but when we sang duets or harmonized together, we created a sonic texture richer than what we were able to create alone. Our voices and songs were like individual strands that, when woven together, created a rope strong enough to be a mooring line.

That practice ended the way all our practices ended: my mom came down the stairs at 9 p.m. humming one of the new songs and called curfew.

We played our first show as The Hush for about thirty people in a basement in Naperville. There are two ways to make people listen: raise your voice, or lower it below everyone else's. As I began "Echo," singing it barely louder than a whisper, the conversation fell to a murmur, and I could feel everyone's gaze focused on me. My voice was a sweet, girlish, airy whisper. I'd never had vocal training, so my voice sounded unpolished and uncontrolled, but it had a pureness and clarity to it, like the ring of a muted wind chime. I sang with the same shades of innocence as I'd sung *row row row your boat* when I was a little kid. As a soprano, I sang in head voice, the notes resonating behind my cheekbones and nose rather than more deeply in my throat or chest. Because of nerves, my voice wobbled off pitch sometimes, but it didn't matter. The audience was silent, listening for every word.

Till that point, I'd sung only in my little songwriting cocoon. At that show, I sang the same way—my energy turned inward, inviting the people in the room to observe the experience, rather than singing *out* to them.

When I was singing, I imagined myself in the scene of the song. I was lost at sea, as though I'd entered a dream. Then, the moment the song ended, I snapped back into being myself, sitting behind a Yamaha keyboard in a carpeted basement in Naperville, Illinois.

Afterward, my high school friends raved. One of them loved

the show so much that she cornered me in the bathroom and insisted on joining the band. "We could be like Fleetwood Mac," she said. "I'll be Stevie and you'll be Christine." After I said no, she gave me the silent treatment. At school on Monday, friends must've been talking about the show because my history teacher, Mr. Kibbs, greeted me saying, "I hear The Hush rocked this weekend!"

Soon, Darren's close friend Chris, who'd been his bandmate in another local group, joined as our bass player and we moved up to VFW halls and community theaters. During sound check, the sound engineers asked me to sing louder and project more, but when I pushed for volume, I sounded like a baby lion trying to roar. Belting also felt like a psychological leap I wasn't ready to make because it would mean taking up space, commanding attention, expressing bigger emotions than I was ready to share in public. So I stuck to the soft-spoken, lullaby-whisper and let my songs be the moments when the crowd could catch their breath between Bob's faster, grittier anthems.

When Chris went to claim a website for our band, many URLs with "Hush" were already taken. TheHushSound.net was the closest, so he bought it and soon designed and screen-printed our first round of T-shirts, which had a big butterfly with "The Hush" written beneath it. After our third show, we found out that a rapper called Hush had trademarked the name, so we dubbed ourselves The Hush Sound to match the website. Our quirky piano-pop musical style made us an anomaly in the Chicago music scene, which was mostly all-male bands playing guitar-heavy, spiky emo music. The boys and I ate the Zombies for breakfast, the Beatles for lunch, and emo records for dinner, then cooked up our own songs using the same musical ingredients.

Having been a fixture in local bands for years, Bob became the de facto leader of our group. Soon after that first show, creative competition began to flare up between us. At one rehearsal, he told me that my songs were pretty, but insisted that I still needed to learn how to write a catchy chorus. I was so miffed that I started referring to him as The Big Bad Bob Mob in my journal: *The Big Bad Bob Mob said my choruses aren't catchy. I'll show him. I'm going to write the best song The Hush Sound has!*

Eileen moved back to Chicago after eighteen months in Connecticut. One night soon after her return, I met her for dinner at TGI Fridays. Her sparkly, feisty teen mischief had graduated into a darker, sharper wit, and her humor was now tinged with sarcasm. She hadn't enjoyed living in Connecticut and was struggling to adjust to her new high school in Chicago. She'd been in a hot and heavy relationship with her new boyfriend and I felt like a goody-two-shoes by comparison. She'd also started taking Adderall and liked how much energy it gave her. Sometimes, she stayed up all night writing stories and drawing cartoons. When I asked her what the stories were about, she said, "How much I hate my stepdad. Ex-stepdad, actually. I don't want to talk about it."

I kept searching for that bubbly version of her. "Remember how you convinced everyone to run nudie cazoodie off the Water Weenie?" I asked. The Water Weenie was a giant hot-dog-shaped raft that hung off the dock at camp. "Yeah," she let out a single *Ha!* "Does that count as child abuse? I probably shouldn't have done that once we were counselors in training," she said.

It felt like there was a wall between us. When I talked about the band and my music, she seemed confused. I had kept my music hidden from her, so the project seemed like a sudden change. When I came home, I said to my mom, "She's different," but I couldn't put my finger on what felt so strange. I made a point in my journal: *Invite Eileen to the next bonfire.* A few weeks blurred by before I had a chance to talk to her again. Then, one day, I was called out of class to the counselor's office.

The counselor handed me the phone and my mom was on the line. "There's bad news," she said, "and I wanted to be the one to tell you." Then, my mom told me that Eileen had died the night before.

"What?! How?" I said, the words clipping in my throat.

"She took her own life," my mom said.

Tears streamed down my face as I gasped for air, unable to understand the news. My counselor brought in one of my close friends for support, and they stayed with me until my mom arrived. As she drove us home, I was stunned, guilt-stricken, a numbness overtaking me from the outside in. I was four days shy of my sixteenth birthday. It was one of those February days where the sky was the color of sheet metal. The landscape looked like a black-and-white movie: naked trees shivered in the cold wind, the frozen highways were dusted with salt, black crows flew through the sky across a monochrome palette. Eileen would never see any of this again.

When I saw her in the open casket at the wake—mortician's makeup on her cold face, blond hair curled up at the ends, hands folded together—I felt the gates of my childhood close behind me. Like a cave explorer, Eileen had carried the lantern into the unknown terrain of adolescence and waved me on once she determined it was safe. I had walked in her footsteps for so many years and never imagined it could end here. She was dressed in her favorite jeans, a leopard print belt, a cardigan, and a watch, still ticking. For months, I woke up in the middle of the night imagining that watch still ticking underground. After the funeral, I began to have difficulty singing, feeling as though something were constricting my throat.

Bob was sympathetic at the first few band practices, but after weeks went by and I still couldn't sing, he took me aside. "You used to be so much more fun," he said. "You can't let this ruin your life."

Weeks after the funeral, I sat on the floor of Eileen's untouched room with her mom. Eileen's dirty laundry was still in the laundry bin, and the sheets she'd been sleeping in were still on the bed. The room smelled so much like her shampoo that I thought she would step out of the bathroom at any moment.

Mrs. Fitzpatrick handed me Eileen's suicide note, found crumpled up in the trash can after the coroner had left. Eileen had written me hundreds of letters and her handwriting was always carefully plotted—curlicued when she was being playful, boxy when she was determined, with an occasional heart dotting a lowercase *i*. But her suicide note was nearly illegible—scratched, manic inkblots, as if she had written it in the back of a speeding car.

Nothing good ever stays in my life, it began. *I've always tried to stay strong on my own but I can't do it anymore. I can't take being alone. I have no one. No one to talk to.*

The language shocked me because Eileen was always surrounded by friends and family who adored her. Her relationship had ended, which had left her feeling isolated, and this loss had dimmed all the other love in her life.

"You were here so often," Mrs. Fitzpatrick said. "What did I . . ."

At first, she couldn't finish the question. She was looking down at her nails, cracked ivory half-moons. These were the same hands that had washed Eileen's hair, cooked her meals, wrapped her birthday gifts, taught her how to write the alphabet.

"What did I miss?" she finally asked. "How could I be so close to her and not see anything?"

"You were a great mom," I said, sensing that she wanted reassurance, but my words felt inconsequential, like leaves that floated down onto the river of her sadness only to be carried away.

If Eileen had cried out for one of us, rather than keeping her pain to herself, would she have died this way? If she had *voiced* on the phone what she'd written in that suicide note, would she have survived? If I had reached out sooner, if I had known what to say that night at dinner, if only, if only, if only.

In school, my mind was elsewhere, turning the word *suicide* over and over, sharp and flat as a knife. My nightmares about Eileen were so chilling that I slept in my mom's room for much of the second half of my junior year.

One day, I left chemistry class crying and went to sit alone in the chapel. A priest came in to check on me, and when I told him what had happened, he said suicide was the worst sin a person could commit. He said he'd pray for her soul, which was surely in hell.

There were no havens, then, where brokenhearted people could weep and wail without shame. Even the church taught that suicide was a sin against God, since it denied the very life He had given you.

Seeking a version of the afterlife outside of Catholicism, I devoured *The Tibetan Book of Living and Dying* and read Raymond Moody's *Life After Life*, which included stories about near-death experiences that described visions of bright lights, feelings of unbearable beauty, lightness, and oneness. Once I'd begun to read about this unseen world, all the frog dissection, French verb conjugation, and who-was-asking-whom-to-prom drama of high school felt tedious.

The transcendentalist writers like Emerson and Thoreau offered me a spiritual framework large enough to hold all that I felt. They wrote that you didn't need an intermediary to reach God; each person had a direct path to the divine through their own intuition. God was most clearly and easily experienced in the natural world.

Searching for clues about what could drive a person to take

their own life, I read Sylvia Plath's journals and the poetry of Anne Sexton, and listened to Elliott Smith's posthumous record on repeat.

I copied the Langston Hughes poem "Suicide's Note" into my journal, in which the metaphor for suicide is "The calm, / Cool face of the river," asking the writer for a kiss. After that, *water* became a metaphor for death whenever I wrote about Eileen, including one song that I named after her:

> *How I'd love to go*
> *Swim with you in death,*
> *But my heavy heart*
> *Won't let me tread.*
> *So, love, I must stay*
> *On the shore.*
> *I am young,*
> *My blood is warm.*

Comforting myself by writing music was how I emotionally survived that loss. I braided together the raw feelings of grief and confusion with a few poems I'd recently been taught in school. For the bridge of Eileen's song, I worked with the line "when youth and blood are warmer" from Robert Herrick's poem "To the Virgins, to Make Much of Time":

> *When blood and youth were warmer*
> *We breathed Summer like the sweet air*
> *We found each other like a mirror.*

We were so optimistic
Wasn't it so easy to be?
We were young and naïve

When we played the song "Eileen" live, audience members would approach me at our merchandise table after the show and share stories about loved ones they'd lost. I was amazed that I could write a song pulled from my journal, and listeners could feel as though it had come from *their* journal.

I could feel myself being catapulted into the adult world at high velocity, and clung to the roots of my childhood. I read in my room on the weekends, cuddled my dog, and hovered near my mom. But I could tell that my sadness was weighing on her.

In the decade and a half before, my mom had lost both her parents, her marriage, and her longtime script-writing and acting mentor who'd been a father figure to her. A neck injury from a previous car accident caused her debilitating, constant pain that she could relieve only by soaking in Epsom salt baths for hours at a time. Her on-and-off heart trouble worsened, and when she dashed off to Santa Fe to see her homeopathic doctor, my dad came to stay in the guest room for a few days.

My dad recited a proverb: "A parent is only as happy as their unhappiest child." Was he empathizing with me and feeling my pain? Or was he asking me to perform happiness to make his and my mom's lives easier? To unburden everyone, I performed happiness. A perfect student, a prolific songwriter, and an everything-to-everyone-people-pleaser had no time to feel sadness. The knot in my throat tied itself so tight that I could barely eat.

I pulled myself together by pretending that I was an actor playing myself. *What would Greta Sunshine do?* She would finish her lyrics, she would practice her piano parts, she would offer the boys snacks at band practice, she would refer to her dog as the Hush Hound.

Within a year, The Hush Sound had twenty songs and we borrowed $2,000 from my dad to record an album. I promised to pay him back when we started selling CDs. He corrected me: "*If* you start selling CDs." He was a lawyer, after all. He needed evidence. A beat later, he smiled. "You just might."

As soon as we started recording with professional equipment, I was finally able to listen to a high-quality recording of my voice. Hearing my voice back through fancy speakers felt like seeing an X-ray of my soul. Because tissue and bone muffle sound waves internally, we can't clearly hear our own voices when we speak or sing. The distance created by the recording stripped away those distortions, leaving me with the true sound of my voice. Listening was both strange and intimately familiar, like seeing a photograph of my face from an angle I'd never been able to find in the mirror. In my voice, I could hear the fireflies of summer camp, the magnolias of my neighborhood, the child-self who rode in circles on her bicycle.

Bob, Darren, and Chris all congratulated me after the first day of my vocal recording. "I can actually hear you now," Chris said, "and you sound beautiful!"

"Nice one, G," Bob said, high-fiving me. When the producers handed me a CD with a bounce of the song so that I could test it out on my car speakers on the way home, I felt like

I was holding the most valuable possession I'd ever touched. We named the record *So Sudden* because of how quickly the vision for the band had coalesced.

We made a music video for "Crawling Towards the Sun" in which we played ourselves, The Hush Sound, being booed off the stage in a school talent show. We donned saddle mustaches and transformed into The Hush Staches, competing again and earning thunderous applause, winning the talent show. We released it on our website.

One day, leaving school, I received a frantic phone call from Bob telling me we'd been asked to open a sold-out show at the Metro for Motion City Soundtrack. The Metro was holy ground in Chicago, the venue where we'd seen all our idols play. The room held eleven hundred people—about ten times the size of any show we'd ever played. Our stage backdrop, which had filled out tiny suburban VFW halls, now looked dinky, barely big enough for a high school bake sale.

A thousand people were at the show, and we sold more than three hundred *So Sudden* CDs, making $3,000 in one night. Days later, I handed my dad an envelope of cash to repay the album loan in its entirety.

After that show, buzz about our band reached Pete Wentz from Fall Out Boy, who invited us to open for them in northern Illinois. A few weeks later, we pulled into the backstage parking lot of the Forest Hills Lodge in Rockford, Illinois, parking my mom's SUV next to Fall Out Boy's shining silver behemoth of a tour bus. Pete swung the door open and invited us in. The bus reminded me of summer camp—bunks stacked atop each other, three on each side, littered with denim jackets, sweatshirts, and sneakers. It smelled like stale pizza and sweat. In the front lounge, Pete said he'd been listening to "Crawling Towards the Sun" on repeat. His thick black eyeliner made him look sleep-deprived.

Of the four bands, I was the only woman on the bill. Backstage, the throng of male musicians wore skinny jeans, studded leather belts, and the emo version of a mop top—overgrown, choppy hair swept mysteriously over one eye. As I took in the scene of all these boys milling about, I wondered, *Is he cute? Is he cute? Is that one cute?*

We set up our equipment and sound-checked before the audience arrived. Once the theater doors opened, I peered out from the side-stage as the room floor filled with Fall Out Boy's fans. They looked like a cult—a giant sea of dyed-black hair and black Fall Out Boy sweatshirts with big white printed hearts. When you unzipped the sweatshirt, the heart was meant to break in half.

They're gonna hate us, I thought, *especially my piano ballads.* My nerves were on fire as Darren counted off the first song, "Crawling Towards the Sun," and I plunked the piano chords. I stared at my hands, not able to bear seeing the audience's reaction.

Thankfully, Bob performed with a confident, visceral energy. He took jerky steps back and forth while strumming to the beat, bobbing his shoulders side to side. My mind repeated,

Don't mess up, don't mess up, don't mess up, which made me so rigid that my body was barely moving, other than my hands. By the second chorus, I peeked up and noticed people in the front row mouthing the words. By the last chorus, even more people were singing. Pete and Patrick Stump, the lead singer of Fall Out Boy, were watching side-stage, nodding their heads.

Next, we played my song "Weeping Willow." It began with one verse that was just my soft voice and piano. *The snow won't stick to the weeping willows,* I sang. Some folks in the front row looked confused, like they were trying to solve an algebra equation in their heads, but when the boys kicked in for the second verse, the audience started moving, shoulders swaying to the beat. By the time we reached the last chorus, people were also singing along. Song by song, chorus by chorus, we won them over. The rest of our set whirled by in a blur. By the end, I was having so much fun that I broke through my shyness and shoulder-danced a little bit behind my keyboard. When we finished, I was so charged up from the crowd's energy that I felt like I could've single-handedly pushed Fall Out Boy's tour bus up a hill.

As we walked offstage, we exchanged sweaty high-fives with the Fall Out Boy guys and Pete told us we were his new favorite band. "You'll probably sell out of T-shirts tonight, but save a couple for us, can you?" he asked.

I hadn't heard much of their music, so I was surprised by what showmen they were. Onstage the band thrashed around at high speed and their mosh pit was a cyclone of flailing limbs—it looked more like an exorcism than a concert. Pete windmilled his bass in circles, then climbed on top of the bass drum and leaped off it ten feet to the ground. Seeing them create such a euphoric pandemonium made me wonder whether our music, too, could excite a crowd like that someday.

At the merch table, someone asked for my autograph for the first time. I reached for the marker and hesitantly printed my name on their arm. When someone asked me to sign a T-shirt, I tried writing my initials in cursive. For the next autograph, I drew a smiley face and wrote GRETA curved upward on either side as the smile.

After the crowd cleared out and we'd sold all our merch, Chris and I went to drop off the T-shirts we'd saved for the Fall Out Boy guys. I was carrying the mostly empty brown paper merch box, and one of the guys from another band said "Nice box" as we passed by.

"That's weird," I said to Chris. "It's just a normal box." Chris explained that *box* was slang for *vagina*. I didn't know if I should be flattered or horrified. I'd been catcalled by strangers but had never been hit on at a close enough range to actually see the person flirting with me.

In Fall Out Boy's dressing room, Andy, their drummer, who had full-body tattoos, asked me if I had a boyfriend.

"No," I said. "I can't even get a prom date."

"Can I go to your prom with you?" he asked, playing.

"I'm seventeen," I said. "How old are you?"

"Twenty-six," he said, "but I'm turning eighteen soon."

Oh. My. God. It was like I'd entered a parallel reality. Suddenly, the same traits that made me invisible to the cool guys at school—my bookishness, my desire to play piano instead of partying, my sexual inexperience—now made me attractive to older male musicians who dug the fact that I was a Catholic school girl. Back in our dressing room, Darren doubled over with laughter and offered to pay me $500 to take Andy to the Benet Academy prom.

When I got home that night, I wrote a six-page journal entry titled BEST! NIGHT! OF! MY! LIFE! Before that night, my journal was equally devoted to school, family, friendships, and the band. After that show, the rest of the journal became devoted exclusively to the band. Days later, Pete Wentz emailed asking to sign us to his record label, Decaydance, an imprint of Warner Records.

Soon, Pete sat at my dining room table having brunch with my parents to persuade them to sign a record deal on my behalf, since I was still a year shy of legal age. Pete promised to take us on tour as an opener, to connect us with the management company that represented Fall Out Boy, and to advertise our band to the best of his ability. When the ink dried, I had committed to a three-album contract. They would do a soft rerelease of *So Sudden* while we wrote and recorded the next one. The stakes for our second record felt dramatically higher than the first. Now, a record label and our new management team, Crush Management, were invested in our success, and my bandmates saw the financial potential. Our manager, Bob McLynn, was a former hardcore musician who had a shaved head, massive biceps, and a big, shining smile. We nicknamed him Mr. Clean.

In September 2005, we went to New York City to play a

showcase at CBGB so that the head of our record label, John Janick, could see us perform. Eastbound on I-90, my heart was fizzing with excitement; I felt like we were driving toward the rest of my life, leaving behind the humdrum routine of high school English and physics. Signing a record contract at my age seemed as rare as winning the lottery. My euphoria was tempered when we took the stage at CBGB and performed for exactly three people: our label boss, my dad, who was in town on business, and my great-aunt, who lived in the city. We had a contract, yes. But an audience outside Chicago? Not quite yet.

While in New York City, I was invited to participate in a photo shoot for a story *Teen People* was doing on up-and-coming teenage musicians. Not knowing what to wear, I'd brought my blue-lace strapless homecoming dress from the previous year. The makeup artist gave me a glamorous, old Hollywood look with dramatic false eyelashes. The hairstylist curled my hair into voluminous waves and used a fan to create a windswept look during the photo shoot. "Tilt your head down to the left, open your mouth slightly, now look up at the lens," the photographer said. I felt stiff, self-conscious, and caked in chemicals, but the photographer grinned and said, "That's your LOOK! There she is!"

The other young artists were bursting with outward confidence, and they all had clever elevator pitches for their music. One woman said she aspired to be "our generation's Janis Joplin." Another said her music "had the rebellious spirit of Alanis Morissette with the pop sensibility of Paramore." Another said she was like "if Britney Spears loved poetry" and made "pop music with soul." When the interviewer asked me what my music sounded like, I just said, "Ummmm, I usually write songs about my dreams."

. . .

In the spring of 2006, we were recording our second album, *Like Vines*. On the first day of tracking lead vocals, I had woken up at 4:30 a.m. to study for a chemistry test. In the afternoon, I walked into the recording studio still wearing my high school uniform—a plaid skirt, a button-down collared shirt, knee-high socks, leather loafers.

My bandmates were gathered in the lounge surrounded by greasy paper bags of burgers and fries. Fall Out Boy's Patrick Stump was producing our record, and Bob and Patrick both had guitars on their laps, punching up one of Bob's choruses. I poured a cup of stale coffee and dug around in the cabinets for snacks. Patrick, noticing my uniform, played a rendition of Billy Joel's "Only the Good Die Young":

> *Come out, Virginia, don't let me wait*
> *You Catholic girls start much too late.*

Then I stood at the microphone in the vocal booth to record the vocals for "Magnolia." It was a sweeping, bittersweet song I wrote as a plea of hope for two girls at my high school who were struggling with depression. One had just been hospitalized for a suicide attempt and another taken out of school for anorexia treatment. The chorus lyric was, "Run where you'll be safe, through the garden gates, to the shelter of magnolias."

Patrick and Sean O'Keefe, another producer, were in the control room behind the big mixing board. I could see them through soundproof glass windows but I couldn't hear them. I sensed they were discussing my voice, and I tried to read their lips but couldn't make out what they were saying. After each take, Sean and Patrick would press the talk-back button to give me feedback.

"Too nasal," Sean said after one take. "Can you sing it breathier?"

I sang a breathier version.

"Too wispy. Can you sing it louder?" he said.

I sang it louder but my voice cracked a little. I didn't know how to belt, and my voice was naturally soft and childlike. I sounded like what I was: a teenager. And a late bloomer at that; I was still a virgin. When they pointed out that certain notes were flat or sharp, I couldn't hear exactly what they meant. I loved the wonky, off-pitch vocal deliveries of John Samson from the Weakerthans, Conor Oberst from Bright Eyes, and Davey von Bohlen from the Promise Ring, but it was clear that they wanted this record to be more polished.

"Greta, can you sing it more like this?" Patrick said, and then sang the line with greater emphasis on the high note of the chorus. I copied him on the next take, though it felt unnatural. I was frustrated by my vocal limitations and felt small and powerless being asked, and expected, to imitate him. Patrick and Sean had made hit records, and I had not. They were the ones controlling the mixing board, choosing which takes made it onto the record, and deciding when we were finished. As a young person who'd had a lucky break, I felt I should act agreeable and be grateful just to be there. But the producers were trying to manipulate my voice in a way that made me uncomfortable.

After several takes of imitating Patrick, I heard a flash of Sean's voice letting out an exhausted sigh and saying, ". . . gonna take forever." He'd accidentally pressed the talk-back button. Eventually, they asked that we try vocal takes word by word, slicing the lyrics into shards. At a point of diminishing returns, Patrick called a break and came into the booth.

"Look, Greta, I know you can do this," he said. "You can sing with your full voice. It's definitely in there. Haven't you ever belted before?"

"Only when I'm joking around," I said. "I don't have that kind of big, belting voice."

"You always sing in your head voice, which is soft and nice but . . . we're gonna need to get some power on this take. You need to sing this one with your balls."

Maybe I was afraid to use my full voice for the same reason I was afraid to express anger or cry in front of people—taking up that kind of space felt unthinkable. I wrote songs that came from tenderheartedness and melancholy, which were meant to be sung softly, not belted.

After six hours, Patrick and Sean sent me home with a few Fiona Apple records, noting how strong and confident her voice was. Back then, my songwriting, my vocal style, and my identity felt inextricably linked. Being asked to sing like other people implied that there was something inherently wrong with my voice and, by extension, something wrong with *me*. After they pointed out flaws in my voice, I could never hear myself sing without coming back to their criticisms.

We recorded the rest of the album in this way, splicing the lyrical lines word by word, until I satisfied their requests. When I listened to the final mix of the album, I couldn't even enjoy the songs that I'd written because all I could hear was how auto-tuned and chopped the vocal takes had been. It gave me a sour feeling, like a layer of cellophane had coated my living, breathing voice.

Afterward, I embarked on a quest to train my voice to be stronger, more agile, and more expressive. I studied the techniques of my idols and scoured replays of my live performances with a hypercritical eye, measuring myself with unrelenting harshness. I started writing darker songs, tinged with anger, as if that would make me seem more mature, and singing with a sultry growl, like an imitation of Fiona Apple.

• • •

In the spring of my senior year, we opened six weeks of Fall Out Boy's arena tour while I finished high school by correspondence. Our guarantee was $50 per night, but it didn't matter because we were going ON TOUR!

It was surreal to do my homework in the catering area, email my teachers from the dressing room, then step onstage to perform for fifteen thousand people. Before that first show in Albany, New York, in March 2006, Mr. Clean told us to move around ten times as much onstage as we used to so that we could connect with the people way up in the nosebleed seats. We exaggerated our movements like he suggested, and performing that way felt like creating a caricature of our band, magnifying our emotions and stage movements.

Surprisingly, performing the first time in a big, echoing arena felt less nerve-racking than some of our smaller, early shows. We were so far from the crowd that I couldn't read their facial expressions. Our songs became booming echoes, projected to the room and beamed back to us. At the smaller shows, I felt like a human connecting with other living, breathing humans. At the arena shows, I felt like a statue being viewed from all sides. I couldn't see people individually, but I could feel thousands and thousands of eyes on me.

The word *confident* comes from Latin *confidere*, meaning "to trust." I was not yet confident in my body, not yet confident in my voice or my stage presence. The only thing I trusted were the songs. I wanted the spotlight and I also wanted to shield myself from its glare.

Backstage, Pete Wentz looked at our humdrum suburban clothes and announced, "You guys should dress like you're in a Wes Anderson movie." The next day, he went thrift shopping on our behalf and brought back 1970s sepia-colored polyester collared shirts for the guys and a pink vintage raincoat for me.

At the merchandise table, our tour manager, Emily, directed

the large swarms of listeners into a line to take pictures one by one. "No hugging. No kissing. No freaky stuff. Say hello. Take a picture. Be nice," she said, over and over. By the end of the first week of that tour, I was dashing off high-speed cursive signatures like a business mogul. People often told me my voice was "cute" or "adorable," which I always received as an insult. It added to my eagerness to train my voice to be stronger, deeper, more powerful.

To navigate from venue to venue, we printed out turn-by-turn directions from MapQuest before we got on the road. We put hundreds of these sheets of paper in a three-ring binder but often had to read maps whenever highways were closed or we got lost. One night early on, I missed a highway exit and Bob ripped into me: "Just because you go to a fancy private school doesn't mean you have smarts in the real world." I let his words hang in the disgusting air of our van, which smelled like Subway sandwiches and oily skin. Back in Chicago, he and I bounced back from conflict because we had breathing room and time apart to cool down, but our friendship started to curdle in the claustrophobia and pressure of the tour.

A week later, after a show in Grand Rapids, Michigan, I took the second night shift of the seven-hour drive to St. Charles, Missouri. Somewhere between Illinois and Missouri, a highway was closed but I was determined to prove that I could find my way without consulting the guys. I wound up making widening circles in the state of Missouri, in the pitch-dark farmland, getting no closer to our destination, while everyone else slept. When Bob blinked awake at 8 a.m., bleary-eyed and disoriented, he said, "Why the hell aren't we in St. Charles yet?"

"Because I don't have street smarts," I said. "Welcome to Hannibal: the boyhood home of Mark Twain!"

Before we left for the tour, I'd wanted to tie a canoe atop our van to take nature adventures on days off, but the boys said no. A week into the tour, when we were blasting our brains with gas station coffee and mainlining Snickers bars to drive twelve-hour overnight shifts, I realized how silly the canoe would've been. We wouldn't pay for a hotel unless we knew we'd be there for four hours or more, so we often slept in Walmart parking lots for a few hours at a time, each of us in one row of the four van rows with one of us on the floor.

Driving all night felt like witnessing a secret, behind-the-scenes version of America. Construction crews tarred the highways, tollbooth operators exchanged change in the pre-dawn, waiters brought waffles and bacon to nocturnal diners, bleary-eyed hotel clerks greeted us at the desk at 5 a.m. As a teenager, lost in the electrifying energy of a concert, I had never considered the twenty-two to twenty-three hours a day that existed beyond the performance. All musicians, I realized, lived in a perpetual state of *in-between*.

The dashboard was covered with hardened used Kleenex—"snot rags," as we called them. We referred to our trusty Ford Econoline E350 van as the Fart Mobile, which was what it became after late-night Taco Bell visits. Every few days, we pulled the Fart Mobile up to a Bank of America and deposited tens of thousands of dollars in cash from our T-shirt and CD sales.

At our show in San Diego, Tim, my eighth-grade boyfriend who'd taught me to play guitar, spent the day backstage with us. He had a day off from his training with the Marines nearby and beamed with pride as he saw me play onstage. Afterward, he asked if I still wanted to honor the marriage contract we'd made.

"Houlihan's napkins are legally binding," I joked.

"We should probably start looking for venues," he smiled and kissed me on the cheek goodbye.

I had no idea this would be the last time I'd see him. Three months later, Tim would die as a result of a drinking incident in the Marines. His organs would be donated to save the life of the father of one of his classmates. Bob and I attended the funeral, but our travel schedule was so demanding that I never truly stopped to grieve. Losing two of my closest companions in such sudden ways brought life's fragility and impermanence into sharp focus in my daily life. I became hyperaware of *lasts* in life, even in mundane moments. As I mourned their losses, a low-level panic crept in, a voice that asked, *Who will I lose next?*

My mom suggested that the best way to honor Tim and Eileen was to embody their best qualities. Every time I did something playful—like the week on tour when, every morning, I grabbed Bob's new modern Japanese eyeglasses off the bedside table before he woke up and hid them somewhere in the room—I thought of Eileen. I honored Tim's supportive warmth and kindness by encouraging and uplifting friends who were shy about their art. "The best songs come to those who keep their instruments close," Tim had said. I kept sleeping with my guitar in bed. It still makes me think of him.

• • •

A month into the tour, in Tacoma, Washington, Chris and I walked around the Tacoma Dome before sound check. The twenty-thousand-person arena echoed like a giant, cold refrigerator while the sound team built the stage and the janitorial team cleaned the floors. Chris said, "I know we're lucky to be here, but doesn't it feel like we should have worked for ten years to earn a tour like this?" Our ascent had taken on a life of its own. The rest of the year had already been booked through with concerts.

After the Fall Out Boy tour finished, I put on my uniform and returned to school to take my finals. The scale had shifted again: suddenly, I felt too big for the halls of my high school. I skipped prom to go on tour in the UK, and when the principal read my name at graduation, he said, "Absent . . . due to being a rock star." My dad and stepmom planned a vacation to Scotland to see us play.

My school friends set off for expensive colleges and I embarked on my own education—crisscrossing the country, playing hundreds of shows, and living packed-as-sardines with the boys in the van, in dressing rooms, in hotel rooms, and on the stage.

I'd always considered myself a sidekick in The Hush Sound—Art Garfunkel to Bob's Paul Simon—but when the *Like Vines* record came out in June 2006, a Chicago paper wrote a story about us, and I was surprised that it was focused on me:

From a shot in her high school yearbook to a shot in *Teen People*, from a performance at the local VFW hall to an opening gig at the UIC Pavilion, success has come quick for Oak Brook resident Greta Morgan Salpeter and her bandmates in The Hush Sound. . . . . To get an idea of The Hush Sound's skyrocketing popularity, the band's MySpace Website has more than 500,000 hits and their current national tour with Panic at the Disco and The Dresden Dolls is sold out at almost every venue from Washington DC to Seattle.

"Getting signed was pretty ironic," Salpeter said. "We were just getting together to have fun and to play the music that we like to hear, and then something like this just fell into our lap."

But the joy of being recognized for my music was often tainted by negative or misogynistic comments. Between late-night fast food and the limitless backstage catering options, I ate a lot of junk on tour. When people commented on our YouTube live videos that I'd been gaining weight, I spiraled into self-consciousness and self-soothed with food. I wound up wearing that pink rain jacket all the time to cover my body on tour, an item that simultaneously said *look at me* and *don't look at me*.

When we performed on a TV show at a local station, the male host asked us during the live taping, "Who's the biggest partier in the band?"

The boys all pointed to me, teasing me with love because I was in fact the prude. Chris said to the host, "She never parties. Yoga is her drug of choice."

The host turned to me and said, "Can you show us a downward dog?"

"Not now," I said. "I'm wearing a dress."

"Isn't that the best way to demonstrate it?" he asked and laughed. We were being filmed and I froze. My face went red, horrified, but I couldn't speak.

I felt powerless over the way I was presented. Nude photos of Pete Wentz had leaked earlier that year online, creating an internet sensation. When our record came out, he re-created one of the photos, holding our CD over his penis. As with everything in our band, we voted on whether to approve the advertisement. The boys approved it, finding it hilarious. I voted no—it felt like a cheap trick—but the ads ran in *Alternative Press* magazine and many other places online. I thought back to the brunch we had with my parents: Pete had, indeed, kept his promise to advertise our album to the best of his ability.

In the late summer of 2007, the Hush Sound guys and I moved to Los Angeles to record our third record, *Goodbye Blues*. We lived at the Oakwoods, a furnished apartment complex that mostly housed child actors and their manager moms. Since we were separated from our families, friends, and hometown, the recording session became an all-encompassing pressure cooker. We lived in a two-bedroom apartment and each room had twin beds, so Bob and I slept parallel to each other the way couples did in television shows in the 1950s.

We all numbed out in different ways, the boys with pot and me on the elliptical machine ninety minutes at a time. Bob and our producer clashed almost daily, and afterward, the producer would ask me, "Can you go fix it?" and send me to console Bob. Bob and I argued constantly over whose songs would find a place on the record. We needed each other, but even more than that, we needed to be *better* than each other.

Our team wanted us to write a hit. The producer paired us up with professional songwriters to "punch up" a few of our demos that had "hit potential." I thought songs were supposed to come from lightning bolts of inspiration and sincere emotional outpourings, so I was shocked and horrified to learn that hit-songwriting was, for many people, like a desk job. Songwriters in countless LA studios churned out songs from nine to five, co-writing with artists, aiming for a No. 1 single.

Many of our labelmates performed on the MTV Video Music Awards that year while we were recording. Mr. Clean promised we'd be up on that stage the following year. The Hush Sound boys and I simultaneously wanted that success, but we were all also totally freaked out about reaching that level. We started self-sabotaging. When our manager suggested that one of my songs needed "a more explosive chorus," we edited in the sounds of World War II artillery from a movie and sent it back.

One night, Patrick from Fall Out Boy took me and Bob out to dinner at Mel's Drive-In diner in Hollywood. When Bob was in the bathroom, I confided in Patrick that I was miserable. The fighting. The pressure. The piercing loneliness I felt, despite being constantly surrounded by the guys. Patrick reminded me how the band had started: we were friends, having fun, making music we loved in the basement, not worried about what would happen next. "Anything you make will be good, whether it's with the guys or on your own," he told me. "You just have to make your relationship with music fun again." But I couldn't figure out how to access that lighthearted spirit the band used to feel together.

On the release of *Goodbye Blues*, our team suggested that I become the front person and that Bob move side-stage. Our bass player, Chris, printed out a golden star with my name in the center and hung it on our dressing room door. I laughed it off, but something felt true: I wanted creative freedom. I was constantly listening to Jenny Lewis's *Rabbit Fur Coat*, the solo record she had made after years of playing in a male/female songwriting duo as part of the band Rilo Kiley. She'd stepped out creatively, telling intimate stories about her life with vivid details and heartaching, torch-song vocal deliveries. With her as my inspiration, I imagined making a solo record, though I didn't feel *quite* ready to go off on my own yet.

Around that time, I learned that Ezra Koenig, the lead singer of Vampire Weekend, was my third cousin through marriage. His extended family had an email chain connecting hundreds of Koenigs across the country, including my grandmother, Lynn. When Grandma Lynn received an email about Vampire Weekend being featured on the cover of *Spin* magazine, she replied to the thread that Ezra wasn't the only musician in the family and she shared my upcoming tour dates.

Before long Ezra and I connected, and he wrote me a kind email about my song "Hurricane." We stayed in touch and sent supportive messages when the other released new records.

• • •

Our *Goodbye Blues* headlining tour was sold out in the summer of 2008. As the band grew in popularity, so did our crew. We were joined by a tour manager, a sound guy, a merch person, and my photographer friend Ani, who came out to document our life on the road. It should've been a joyful victory lap, but the tour gods cursed us one week after another. Our bus broke down repeatedly in the Southwest and turned into a 105-degree sauna. The power went out during our first song at one show and the event had to be canceled. In Yuma, Arizona, Border Control found marijuana on our bus and my bandmates received huge tickets. Bob and I fought in a tug-of-war for creative control of the band. Instead of naming our actual conflict, we engaged in looping, marathon arguments. He dismissed my favorite Elliott Smith songs as "boring background music." Days later, in a petty move, I left a bunch of college applications open on my computer, flaunting my privilege and opportunity.

One day, Bob pulled two cartons of my broccoli sprouts from the tour fridge and replaced them with his leftover pizza. "You can't take up the entire fridge, Greta," he said.

"You guys use the entire front and back lounge coolers for alcohol and I don't drink any of that. I deserve more fridge space."

"That's not fair," he said. My skin went magma-hot with fury. I stood up and screamed, "Do not touch my fucking broccoli sprouts!" It was the first time I'd ever yelled on my own behalf. Bob backed away slowly as if I were a grizzly bear.

The guys and I tried to diffuse tension with humor that

summer. We'd all loved Amy Winehouse's *Back to Black* record and pored over interviews with her. In one interview that we watched together, she said: "I was talking to my producer, Mark Ronson, and I told him, 'My dad's trying to make me go to rehab and I keep saying no, no, no.' Mark said, 'Amy, that's brilliant. Put it in a song!'"

"Put it in a song" became the catchphrase of the summer. When one of our crew members stepped out of the bathroom at a venue and said, "That spicy Thai food gave me explosive diarrhea," Bob dipped into a British accent and chimed, "That's brilliant. Put it in a song!" One day, when I was reading a *National Geographic* issue about the deep sea, I gasped and said, "Did you know jellyfish are immortal? And blobfish don't have any bones!" Chris said, "Greta, that's brilliant," and then they all chimed together, "Put it in a song!" Unfortunately, we never had *quite* enough humor to heal the deeper conflicts.

As Bob and I continued to fight, the merch table became an oasis of social connection. I asked our listeners so many questions about their lives that our merch guy called me Barbara Walters Junior. What were they afraid of? What did they long for? What gave their life meaning? What were their predictions for the future? Year after year, the same people would show up at the merch table and update me on what had happened to them in the interim. I posed for photos with everyone who wanted them, even as venue employees tried to kick everyone out.

I felt a piercing romantic longing on that tour. I'd been single for much of the Hush Sound's career, never in one place long enough to start a relationship. At age twenty, I deeply longed for the kind of creatively collaborative partnership I'd seen modeled by Joan Didion and John Dunne, Frida Kahlo and Diego Rivera, Johnny Cash and June Carter.

Nearing the end of the tour, I'd been itchy for weeks and blamed it on stress and sweltering heat. On a day off, Chris offered us psychedelic mushrooms, hoping to create a new harmony between all of us. After taking the mushrooms by a peaceful body of water in Needles, California, I scratched my itchy scalp, then glanced at my hand. There, in the glinting sunshine, two lice writhed beneath my fingernail. In my mind's eye, the lice looked like giant black alarm clocks with flashing red eyes. I thought they might climb into my ears and eat my brain.

Ani hadn't taken mushrooms, so she took charge. We hopped on bikes and she led me to a pharmacy in town where we bought all the lice shampoo they sold. When the total was $66.66, I looked at her as if I'd seen a UFO land in the canned food aisle. "Don't freak out," she said, and added a chocolate bar.

At the Holiday Inn, I tied my thick, wavy, waist-length hair in a ponytail and cut it off below my shoulders. I lathered the poisonous shampoo on my scalp and waited twenty minutes. There was a *Law & Order* marathon on television, so we listened to detectives solve rape and murder cases while I combed hundreds of tiny bugs out of the nest of my hair with a metal-tooth comb. Exhaustion and depression were as thick as the heat that summer. Every time a detective said, "We're looking for a missing girl," I felt an echo that I'd gone missing, too.

My best hometown friend, Samantha, called. She was at Lollapalooza with our other Chicago friends watching Phantom Planet, one of our favorite bands. "Wish you were hereeeeeeee!" they said, holding the phone up so I could hear the band playing.

"I wish I was, too," I said, tears falling down my face.

At that moment, all I wanted was to be a normal twenty-year-old, home from college for the summer, unsure about the future, dumb with joy at my favorite band's concert.

In *The Beatles Anthology* documentary, George Harrison says, "It was great that we wrote hits and made so much money right away because that's how we realized money wouldn't make us happy." He recalled that in the madness of Beatlemania, the fans "gave their money and they gave their screams. But the Beatles kind of gave their nervous systems, which is a much more difficult thing to give."

Living my dream of being a professional musician at such a young age showed me that commercial success does not guarantee happiness. In my case, it brought deeper personal lows and harsher self-criticism than before.

• • •

At the end of 2008, The Hush Sound was offered another three-album contract from our record label with twice the money as our first deal. Our manager, Mr. Clean, pitched a new angle: "Amy Winehouse. Duffy. You know why they are successful? They're VINTAGE. All four of you can sing. Let's turn you into a barbershop quartet. We're gonna make you guys VINTAGE. People want VINTAGE!"

After that conversation, our bass player, Chris, quit; he had been my closest friend in the band. We had two tours left—one in Japan, and a US tour opening for OneRepublic—so we hired a replacement for Chris. After a rehearsal in downtown Chicago, Bob and I went for a walk and I told him that I couldn't play in the band much longer. The constant tension had sapped all my creative energy. My spirit felt fried to a crisp. Bob insisted that we were better together and that we could breathe new life into the project. He said that we'd never *really* made the record we were capable of making and that we should try harmonizing entire songs the way the Everly Brothers did. I agreed that we hadn't reached our creative potential, but depression had settled over me like a lead bodysuit, and I worried that staying in the band would mean sabotaging my mental health even more. I held my ground.

Stepping off the plane at the Tokyo airport arrivals terminal we were met by a wave of our Japanese listeners offering gifts and thank-you cards. Witnessing the band's impact so far from home, with people who didn't speak our language, brought up a deep conflict within me. What if my luck with The Hush Sound was a once-in-a-lifetime experience? Though I dreamed of making music on my own, I doubted whether my voice could carry an entire album.

Touring without Chris was hard. He'd been the one person in the band with whom I always felt safe expressing myself.

Still, I recognized what an extraordinary gift my success was. The women in my family, and so many women in history, had been punished for expressing their emotions. There I was, on the other side of the world, sharing mine onstage.

We played one last show at the Metro in Chicago. My mom sat in the stage-right balcony, her smile shining down at us. My dad sat in the stage-left balcony, wearing his custom-made Hush Sound baseball cap, which had *HUSH* on the front and *SOUND* on the back. They both seemed so proud, even as they supported my choice to step away from the band.

I sang my heart into every word, now belting to the back of the room. It was heartbreaking to sing those songs live not knowing whether we'd ever perform them again. After the encore, we all stood at the front of the stage, arm in arm, a wave of applause filling the air. I'd been a prism capable of many possible expressions of light, but my creative spirit had been refracted into a single color with this band for four years. As the stage went dark, the lights and the amps went silent, and something deeper within myself went silent as well.

After that show, Bob gave me a letter that read: "When I met you, you were a shy little girl bursting with creativity. I've watched you become a woman who is confident in her abilities. I've watched you learn how to stand up for yourself . . . I'm so, so sorry that I was one of the reasons you had to learn that."

Two days later, The Hush Sound announced its indefinite hiatus.

FOUR

I COULD DESTROY YOU, BUT I WON'T WASTE MY TIME

AFTER THE HUSH SOUND BROKE UP, I SPENT A YEAR LIVING IN Los Angeles and couldn't find my footing. In 2010, I returned to Chicago and started a sugary, summery power pop band called Gold Motel. I also decided to ditch my last name, Salpeter, and chose to use Greta Morgan, my first and middle names. I wanted the band name to have the same initials as me, a subtle signal that I was the creative force behind the project. Gold Motel felt like a metaphor for a never-ending road trip, a kind of Kerouac-esque, unbridled freedom.

I moved back into my mom's house in the suburbs to save up money to record an album. My Gold Motel bandmates were a dream team: Three came from a local band called This Is Me Smiling, whom the Hush Sound guys and I worshipped.

Our other bandmate, Eric, wrote and played guitar in a string of Chicago bands that I'd loved. I envisioned us as a Chicago supergroup, with me as the lead singer carrying every song. The songs we wrote sounded like the sensory experience of peeling an orange—bright, fresh, effervescent, pure summer. "Beach Blanket Bingo with Blondie" is how a listener once described our music. I imitated Debbie Harry and Chrissie Hynde from The Pretenders, leaning into the nasal-bright sound of my voice, while our two guitar players built driving, rhythmic, Strokes-esque guitar parts beneath.

Gold Motel changed my life in two major ways: Our guitar player and engineer, Dan Duszynski, taught me basic recording skills so I could track vocals alone without anyone nitpicking me and home-record my own in-progress song demos. Also, Eric introduced me to his cousin, Eddie.

When Eddie and I met, he was also twenty-one, studying screenwriting and directing at Columbia College downtown. He always kept a pencil behind his ear, like he was ready to receive the next great idea. He was a former cross-country runner, six-feet-two and thin, with deep brown puppy dog eyes, Irish freckles on his cheeks and eyelids, copper-brown hair, and a laugh that felt like sunshine on sand. His S sounds had an ever-so-slight whistle to them, barely noticeable but charming.

Eddie offered to direct the music video for "Perfect in My Mind," a sun-drenched, upbeat retro-pop song about seeking comfort in love despite distant impending doom. I immediately volunteered to do all the prop shopping with him so we could spend time together. I sent him a photo reference of a girl in a room full of balloons, and when I arrived at the set, he'd created the exact scene I'd envisioned. But he was always so professional and even-keeled that I thought he must not like me as much as I liked him. When he was behind the camera, I felt his eyes on me and wondered whether he thought I was beautiful. I fantasized about kissing him many times and worried my face was giving me away.

Weeks later, he hosted a *Mad Men*–themed party. Everyone was dressed in 1960s attire and drinking Manhattans from highball glasses. When I watched him dance with a woman in an emerald-green dress, I thought, *Shit. I really like him. But he obviously doesn't like me back if he's dancing with her.*

Weeks later, I invited him over to my mom's house and admitted I had feelings for him. In my childhood basement, we shared one of those kisses that feels like being bolted back to life with a defibrillator. He told me he wouldn't have made a move if I hadn't done so first because he was too intimidated by me.

Later that winter there was an arctic chill in Chicago and he hosted another party at his apartment. After everyone left, the song "Message to Pretty" by Love played on the stereo as we fell into bed together, dizzy and drunk. The singer sang,

I go through life searching, trying to find the one . . .

It was so early in our relationship, but when I heard that lyric, I *knew* Eddie was the one. The next line came as a surprise:

I go slip slip, you go slip slip away . . .

We were making out with such intensity that I worried his cheap futon would break. "Don't go slip slip away," I said, pulling him closer.

"I won't go slip slip away," he said.

We had drunk, dizzy dreams, sleeping with our heads on the same pillow. In the morning, the empty streets were iced over and we skated down the sidewalks in our shoes, holding each other for balance, our breath like little clouds in front of us, our eyes stinging from cold, the warmth of new love glowing from our bodies.

Our relationship became a never-ending chorus of *have you ever . . . ?* and *what if we . . . ? Have you ever seen* Wings of Desire *by Wim Wenders? What if we listened to every Beatles record in chronological order? Have you ever heard that story about Robert Johnson trading his soul to the devil?*

Eddie and I watched *Eames: The Architect and the Painter,* a film about the husband-wife design team Charles and Ray Eames, who had created the iconic Eames chair. They also collaboratively designed homes, toys, short films, and even splints for World War II veterans. Their studio motto was "Take your pleasure seriously."

Eddie said, "I want our partnership to feel like that. Minus his affair at the end." This was finally the kind of love story I'd spent many years fantasizing about—two artists in love, mirroring the best in each other, sharing our in-progress work, challenging each other to be bolder and braver. We channeled the Eameses' spirits, collaborating on his short films and my record covers and music videos.

I'd naïvely assumed Gold Motel would achieve the same level of success as The Hush Sound. Then, cue the crickets: Gold Motel played to nearly empty clubs everywhere outside of Chicago.

When we went on tour, the guys and I slept five to a room in supercheap hotels. Showers dribbled brown rust-water, one bathroom door had a fist hole punched through it, there were cigarette burns on too many bedside tables to count, and the bedspreads were so grimy that under UV light they'd probably look like crime scenes. In one hotel, I pulled back the blinds to discover that there wasn't even a window: the room was a solid, concrete box. Gold Motel? More like Mold Motel.

One East Coast tour culminated with a show at the Holiday Inn in Altoona, Pennsylvania, at which all eight audience members talked through the entirety of our set. Afterward, Eric suggested that, when it came to Gold Motel going on tour, the "juice was not worth the squeeze." I found myself in a situation nearly identical to the years before: unhappy, trapped in a tour van with a bunch of boys. Worse yet, I was draining my savings by funding our recordings and tours.

Gold Motel amicably broke up in the summer of 2012 and we all ventured off to other creative projects. Eddie moved to Los Angeles for grad school at the American Film Institute and I moved there to join him. We rented the upper level of a duplex that belonged in a children's storybook: the chimney was the shape of a gnome's hat and the front yard had a massive century plant with silver-green, sword-shaped arms. Perched on a hillside overlooking the San Gabriel Mountains, our bedroom was peaceful as long as the windows were shut. When we slid our patio door open, the rumbling-thrumming-bustling-beeping of the highway below flooded in and the black dust of exhaust settled on our dresser and desk.

Los Angeles felt like a collective fever dream of people bringing their wildest imaginings into life. Everyone we met was in pursuit of a verging-on-delusional ambitious dream. At any coffee shop, you'd see a half dozen writers punching up screenplays, hear models meeting with managers, eavesdrop on directors and actors talking about their new projects. One writer friend encouraged me to follow her rule, which turned out to be a common practice in that town: "Never lunch alone." She said that networking every day was the path to making professional dreams come true. The word *networking* creeped me out; it felt like the evil twin of *connecting*.

Over Sunset Boulevard, giant billboards of smiling starlets with airbrushed skin and teeth white as moons towered over rows of tents where the city's unhoused slept. In this land of perpetual sunshine, I measured the seasons by the changeover of the television and movie billboard ads. Summer blockbuster season. Emmy nomination season.

In Chicago, I'd become a big fish in a small pond, but coming to Los Angeles, I wondered whether my voice would cut through the high density of other artists and indie singers like me. By the time we were twenty-four, Eddie's screenwriting career was ascending at a meteoric rate and I felt like a washed-up wunderkind, creatively wrung out by making five records with two bands.

"I can't play with a bunch of men anymore," I complained one night in bed. "I want to make something that sounds like *me.* Something they don't get a vote on. I don't want to be responsible for anyone's financial well-being but my own."

I wanted to access the free-flowing creativity I'd felt in my early days writing songs. Eddie suggested that I home-record new songs myself, exactly the way I wanted, and release them anonymously.

"Anonymously?" I asked.

"To get a fresh start in a different scene," he said.

A few days later, I saw a coyote walk out of the woods, and the phrase "Springtime Carnivore" popped into my head. I decided to follow Eddie's suggestion and release under that moniker, without my name attached.

I rented a twelve-by-twelve-foot windowless, concrete rehearsal space and plastered every inch of wall space with colorful postcards and posters I'd collected on tour. I'd arrive at 8 a.m. with a thermos of coffee, then write and record new songs for a few hours, and leave without remembering quite how it happened, as though I'd been in a trance. I was *playing* again, treating music like an experiment. I wanted each Springtime Carnivore song to feel like a shimmering, retro-pop daydream. I channeled my love for '60s and '70s hits, particularly the Motown sound and garage-rock girl groups, by writing sweet, sing-along melodies. But then I subverted the recordings with unexpected sounds and synths, adding layers that felt haunting and strange.

Eddie had encouraged me to reach out to all the artists, filmmakers, and musicians in our extended circle who seemed interesting. That's how I became friendly with Katy Goodman, the bassist of early aughts garage-rock girl group Vivian Girls and lead singer in the band La Sera. Katy had fiery red hair and armfuls of tattoos, and I knew I wanted to be her friend when she closed her eyes and recited thirty digits of pi at a party. She was as passionate about physics and computer science as she was about songwriting. After a few friend dates, Katy and I started playing music together, which was a revelation: our jam sessions were an easy blend of laughter, therapy, and almost telepathic musical communication. We would hike, then jam for a few hours at the rehearsal space, then refuel with California-style veggie bowls, then start all over the next day.

Eddie was my biggest cheerleader, amplifying my creativity and encouraging me to be weirder and bolder, to experiment outside of my usual "square" song structures. He was also our house DJ, turning me on to obscure records I'd never heard, valuing strangeness and distinctiveness above all in art. After we listened to a score by Bernard Herrmann from a Hitchcock film, I experimented with electric string samples. When Eddie played a psychedelic garage-rock compilation called Nuggets, I distorted and fuzzed out my drum sounds the same way. When he played the song "Come Wander with Me," an eerie ballad from the *Twilight Zone* episode of the same name, I was inspired to write a few cinematic interludes on the record.

I played guitar, piano, and drums and then asked Chris from The Hush Sound, who was also living in LA, to record bass. I was overjoyed to collaborate with Chris again in a playful, low-stakes atmosphere. On the first single, "Collectors," I obscured my voice with distortion and reverb to hide myself. To experiment with having a true fresh start, I wanted my voice to be so hidden that even a devoted listener of Gold Motel or fan of The Hush Sound wouldn't recognize it.

Eddie spent a week creating a music video for "Collectors" and hadn't let me see any of it. When it was done, he closed our blinds and pressed "play" on his desktop computer. A montage of vintage photographs flickered in sequence to the beat of the song. Kids frozen mid-dive above a shining lake. A blues duo performing onstage. Red velvet shoes on the feet of schoolgirls. A circle of cigarette smoke leaving red lips. A close-up of a passionate make-out. An elderly couple holding hands on a train. A starry sky above a cabin. The images pulsed with aliveness. It felt like a film montage where a person relives their entire life in one flash. When the video finished, I smothered him with kisses. It was the best gift anyone had ever given me.

Eddie said, "Journalists and record label executives receive a gazillion boring-ass emails every day. We need to write something mysterious to get their attention." He read what he'd written:

I am a traveler and my highways are circuit boards leading to you. You don't know me, but long ago in another age we dined together in a ballroom in Versailles. I was the girl in the green evening gown and the shattered glass slippers. You kissed my hand. We were lovers once. We met in the park; on a pier; in the first-class cabin of the *Titanic*. We sank with the ship. I have written songs about all this and other things, too. I hope you enjoy. Sincerely, Springtime Carnivore.

I loved it.

The release was terrifying and exhilarating. Eddie watched as I emailed two dozen blogs. We spent the day co-working in the bedroom, him editing a script at the desk, me playing guitar on the bed, while we waited for replies. Within hours, I received a message from a blog wanting to spotlight the project. Minutes later, Eddie read from his computer, "Holy shit! Vimeo just put the video on the homepage as a staff pick!" Once the video was on the homepage, it started receiving hundreds of views, then thousands of views. A popular blog called *Line of Best Fit* emailed me asking to feature the video. *Oh my god*, I thought, *Springtime Carnivore is going to work!*

When Eddie and I made love that afternoon, I could barely stop smiling. At dinner that night, he cheered me, clinking our glasses together, and said, "Told you so," with the opposite tone of how people usually mean it.

• • •

In 2013, Eddie directed a music video for Johnathan Rice, the partner of Jenny Lewis, the songwriter whose records had inspired me to go solo. That summer, they invited us over for a Fourth of July party. In the years since I'd become a fan of hers, I continued to read all her interviews and to admire her songs. Her storytelling ability was so keen and bright-minded—she could manage to be clever, soulful, and coy all in one verse. She was a smart person's bombshell—a razor-sharp lyricist who wore the shortest and sparkliest shorts you'd see onstage outside of Las Vegas. I'd read a feature about the architecture of her home in Studio City, nicknamed "Mint Chip" for its green and brown exterior and the stained glass ice cream window. Now, in a surreal moment, Eddie and I were walking up the steps, passing the glowing ice cream window.

Jenny opened the door wearing a white summer dress, smiling, her hair in a loose braid, and offered us Pimm's cups. "Eddie, I've heard so much about you!" she said and then introduced herself to me. "Johnathan, Eddie and Greta are here!" she yelled toward the kitchen. Johnathan was shirtless, wearing a bright green swimsuit, pressing tortillas from scratch, the balls of masa flour laid out in rows on the counter.

I admitted that I didn't realize it was a pool party and hadn't brought a swimsuit. "Got you covered," Jenny said. I overheard Johnathan saying the same thing to Eddie in the living room— "got you covered."

Jenny guided me into the extra bedroom, where a handful of stage outfits were laid out on a twin bed. The red dress she'd worn on the cover of her *Rabbit Fur Coat* record, the one I'd listened to nonstop in my Hush Sound days, was hanging in her open closet. Her gold Wurlitzer, which she played onstage with Rilo Kiley, was in the corner, unplugged. I picked a 1960s baby blue swimsuit with a white stripe print. When I walked out to the pool, Jenny said, "Dang girl, that looks great on you." The swimming pool was a glowing green orb, the shape of a kidney bean. Katy and her boyfriend, Todd, arrived and sat poolside eating tacos. Ferns grew wild up the hillside and cactuses hung from the patio. This felt as close as I'd ever come to the parties I'd seen photos of in Laurel Canyon's 1960s glory days, hosted by Joni Mitchell or Mama Cass.

I played it cool, mostly listening. But when Jenny told a

spa-day horror story about a woman pressuring her to invest in a pyramid scheme while they were both naked in a sauna, I chimed in. "She Lyndon B. Johnsoned you," I said.

"She did what?" Jenny asked.

"I heard that Lyndon B. Johnson used to invite people into his bathroom while he was on the shitter to persuade them into political decisions. If you make someone uncomfortable enough, they'll give in."

"She LBJ-ed me!" she said, laughing.

Afterward, Jenny went into the music room and started playing drums. "Are you summoning us?" I said, as I walked in and sat at the piano and started playing along to her beat. Katy came in and started playing bass. "Katy, can you play one of your songs?" Jenny asked. Katy and I played her song "All My Love Is for You," which we'd just learned at practice. Then Jenny said, "Greta, can you play one of your songs?" Katy had just learned my song "Name on a Matchbook," so we played it with Jenny on drums. Afterward, Jenny told me that the chorus would be stuck in her head. She even sang it back to me. *Jenny Lewis just sang my own song back to me. What world am I living in?*

When we walked back into the living room, Johnathan was sleepily leaning his head on Eddie's shoulder, both of them increasingly tipsy.

"I Will Dare," Eddie said.

Johnathan said, "Color Me Impressed."

Eddie said, "Achin' to Be."

Their conversation made zero sense.

Jenny said, "When Johnathan starts debating the best Replacements songs, that means it's bedtime."

As we said goodbye around 2 a.m., Jenny hugged me and said, "Come back sometime, you two."

Cuddled in bed at home with Eddie, I was giddy. "Can you believe I just jammed with Jenny Lewis?" I said.

"Right where you belong, baby," he said.

Then, in a sleepy, slurring voice, he said, "Can't Hardly Wait."

"Can't hardly wait to go back to another party at Jenny's house?" I asked.

"'Can't Hardly Wait' is officially the best Replacements song," he said, and passed out.

Closing my eyes, a surge of excitement overtook me. I felt that I'd finally landed in the right place at the right time with the right songs.

• • •

Springtime Carnivore became a musical *Room of One's Own*. I was overwhelmed by my love of making music again. Within a week of the "Collectors" video release, a record label from Portugal emailed asking whether it could release a seven-inch on vinyl. Within a month, I'd been offered a generous record deal with Autumn Tone, a Los Angeles–based subsidiary of Anti-, which released the records of many of my favorite bands.

Another one of my musical heroes, the songwriter/producer Richard Swift, signed on to produce a few songs, so in the winter of 2013, I flew up to Cottage Grove, Oregon, to record with him. As a solo artist, I was thrillingly free to collaborate with whomever I wanted without having to run every decision by bandmates.

Richard insisted that we start every recording session with "art time." The first day, we spray-painted a mannequin silver and glued a mosaic on its chest while listening to a playlist we'd made to inspire our recordings. We hodgepodged collages from vintage magazines, and when I put glitter on my collage, he called me Glitter Morgan, a nickname that stuck. When I asked for his advice for making my home recordings sound better, he said, "Don't learn too much. Trust your ears and intuition. Let there be mystery. Just turn the dials till it feels right."

He pulled out a $10,000 Neumann microphone and a cheapo $20 mic from RadioShack and suggested that we do a blind test. I recorded the song on each microphone and then went back to the control room. He played them back and asked which sound I preferred. "The first one," I said. "RadioShack it is!" he said, and we used that mic for the rest of the songs.

When the first Springtime Carnivore record was released, journalists compared my singing to June Carter and Neko Case, which felt like a huge sign of growth—my voice was maturing into a more complex sound, capable of telling different kinds of stories. "Name on a Matchbook," my homage to the Motown melodies of the Supremes and Tammi Terrell, which I'd written and tracked at my rehearsal space, became my most licensed song of all time, eventually landing in dozens of films and TV shows.

Some of my other favorite artists, like the Zombies and Father John Misty and of Montreal, invited me to open for them on tour. When I performed, I always focused on the enjoyment and emotion of the songs while onstage, but afterward, I watched live videos from the shows and nitpicked the expressiveness, strength, and pitch of my voice. The ballad "Other Side of the Boundary" was a benchmark for that, since it was always a solo performance that used my entire range, high into the upper registers for the big-belted chorus. After playing the Horseshoe Tavern in Toronto in early 2015, I rewatched one performance. I watched myself singing, while a number of people in the audience chatted as they drank.

> *Every time I ever tried,*
> *Walking to the edge,*
> *My tired heart would compromise and*
> *I would miss my chance*
> *But I will run now,*
> *I will run now,*
> *Until I see,*
> *The other side of the boundary*

Watching the performance, I thought that, although my voice sounded strong and powerful, it now lacked softness, emotional inflection, and dynamics. I was hitting every line with the same emotional intensity the whole way through. Ironically, the song was about breaking free from fear and self-doubt, yet there I was analyzing every note, unable to step beyond the boundary of my own inner critic.

• • •

Around that time, I peered over Eddie's shoulder as he watched tapes of dozens of beautiful female actors auditioning for the lead role in his first full-length film. They had porcelain skin, high cheekbones, bee-stung lips, bodies like '90s supermodels.

He cast an actor named Emily to play Karen, and on the day I visited the set in Palmdale, California, Emily was filming a sex scene with the male lead. The crew and I stood silently as the two actors tumbled on the bed, and I watched Eddie watch the monitor. My blood bubbled hot, a pang of primal jealousy. In the hotel afterward, I asked Eddie if the character of Karen Bird, named after his mother, was his ideal woman. Karen Bird didn't have a strong sense of inner authority. She camouflaged her desires into the leading man's life, joining his madman dream of driving across the country and attempting to assassinate Elvis.

"You are my ideal woman," Eddie said. "Being around you is like standing near the ocean. You're the most calming person I've ever met." Was *calming* what I wanted to be? Would that be enough to keep him?

Months after the film's completion, it was denied at Sundance and the other major festivals, which was Eddie's first big heartbreak. His hypochondria, formerly a background operation in our life, entered the foreground. He started grinding his teeth at night and developed a nervous tic, clicking his tongue between his teeth like a little alarm clock of anxiety. One night, he woke up at 3 a.m. having a panic attack; I held my hand on his sweaty back and coached him through slow, deep breaths.

On the internet, he searched things like:

Sudden death 27 year old man
Can't sleep foot tingles Parkinson's?
Lungs feel cold . . . cancer?
Freckle on finger . . . cancer?

Unwilling to explore therapy or meditation, he ran the two-mile Silver Lake Reservoir loop many times a day to wear himself out.

"Why did these people give me so much money?" he complained one night. "I feel like such a failure. They should've known better than to let me do this." A thick gloss of irony overcame him, a shield against vulnerability. He added a bio on his website: EDDIE O'KEEFE: HOLLYWOOD PHONY.

Meanwhile, Springtime Carnivore was blossoming. I spent my days writing and recording at the rehearsal space, but as I crossed the threshold back into our home, I dialed down my creative joy to match his mood. I missed the man who had kept the pencil behind his ear.

"Let's have a baby," Eddie suggested over dinner one night. He'd recently read an interview with a famous comedian who claimed that he became "a *real* writer" only after having children, since it altered his perspective of the world.

"With what help?" I asked. "And what money?"

"You could still go on tour," Eddie said.

"How would I raise a newborn on tour?" I asked. "I'm not Beyoncé. We can't afford a nanny."

"We would figure it out," Eddie said. "Maybe my mom could come help while you're on tour."

I had just turned twenty-seven and my record label had just renewed our contract for a second record. I sensed that having a baby would force me to press "pause" on my touring career.

One day, when I was deep-cleaning our kitchen, Lucinda Williams's "Side of the Road" came on. In it, she describes a scene in which she steps out of her car for a moment, knowing that her partner is there but also wanting to be alone. *If only for a minute or two, I want to see what it feels like to be without you,* Lucinda sang. Her words poured out of my own heart.

In Eddie's extended family, the only way you left your partner was if you were being carried away by the coroner. The vital signs of our relationship were still strong: sex every other day, date nights, relaxing in each other's arms listening to records before bed. My parents called him *Steady Eddie.* When he suggested we should move to a certain place in ten years, I was unfazed. *Forever* felt like it was always there for us, stretched out like an endless road. We had just moved into a peachy-pink 1926 craftsman cottage together, which we nicknamed the Pink House, a spacious upgrade from the Silver Lake duplex.

The author Rachel Cusk wrote that when people marry young, "everything grows out of the shared root of their youth . . ." After nearly six years in our partnership, the root of our relationship was so deep that it felt impossible to pull up. That is, until I met Everett Francis.

• • •

Everett was famous for his whiskey-soaked, bleeding-heart Americana ballads and *infamous* for leaving scathing voicemails on the machines of music journalists who wrote bad reviews about him. He was producing a record for some friends who had invited me to play keyboards on the album. I arrived at his studio, Warlock, which was like a dreamworld purgatory in a David Lynch film—green and black checkered floors, red velvet walls, vintage typewriters scattered everywhere, unfinished lyric sheets on the surfaces of desks and shelves, and rare guitars hanging from wall mounts. On the *Cosmic Meadow* album cover, he'd been a stud, but now his leather jacket looked one size too small, giving the impression of a forty-something man dressed up as a teenager. The silhouette of the *Cosmic Meadow* version of him had to be hidden somewhere inside this one.

While I tracked the piano and synthesizer parts, I felt that animal sense of being watched—a bunny nibbling grass, spotted by a wolf. I could feel his eyes on my breasts, my thighs, my hands. To break the tension between takes, I asked the least romantic question possible: "So, who's your favorite president?"

"The more important question," he said, squinting as he looked into my eyes, "is who are *you*?"

He sat next to me on the piano bench and, before the next take, placed his damp palm on the back of my hand to guide it to a higher octave. Shocked by the forwardness of his touch, I jolted away.

"I'm sorry," he said, "I didn't mean to scare you. I swear I'm not a werewolf."

Who swears they're not a werewolf other than a werewolf? I wondered. He backed away into the live room and, with exaggerated warmth, said, "My favorite president is Lincoln."

After watching me play multiple instruments, he took me aside and suggested that I audition for the new lineup of his band. I'd heard from friends that he paid his bandmates $4,000 a week. Life-changing money. I found myself typing my contact information into his phone.

• • •

Here's how to stay in love with your partner: magnify their strengths. Here's how to fall out of love with your partner: magnify their flaws. The Pink House became less charming as it underwent a major overhaul by an electrician named Prince, who drilled and hammered at what seemed like all hours, appearing through holes in the drywall. One day when I opened my closet, Prince was peeking down from a giant hole in the ceiling. In the middle of the night, Eddie joked that Prince might be hiding under our bed, about to pop out the moment we fell asleep. Without AC, the house became an unbearable sauna during the day, and the incessant barking of our landlords' dogs next door drove us insane.

Meanwhile, Everett texted me from his air-conditioned mansion in the Hollywood Hills. He said I reeked of goodness and that he loved the way I stood up straight, as though I was always looking into the future. He told me that he'd been surrounded by intelligent and beautiful women his whole life but that he felt such an intense attraction that it was hard to be in the room together. After listening to Springtime Carnivore, he told me that I was the best-kept secret in rock and roll.

As I walked around the neighborhood reading these messages, my face burned hot with excitement. It felt like a greenhouse full of flowers had erupted within me, blooms pressing up against the glass.

I typed back, "Talking to you feels like finally seeing a starlit sky after a lifetime in light-polluted cities."

He said that the only reason I wasn't more successful was because nobody had ever captured my songs the right way and he asked if he could produce my record. He told me that I was the next Joni Mitchell and he needed to be part of it.

This guy was a field of red flags. On social media, he publicly praised another female songwriter my age, with equally hyperbolic flattery. When I inquired about whether or not they were dating, he FaceTimed me.

"Do you think we would be this attracted to each other if we were in the right relationships?" he asked. My mind drifted back to the Lorrie Moore story "How to be an Other Woman," in which a woman discovers she's not the other woman but the *other other* one. *He has a harem*, I thought. But the glow of his spotlight was intoxicating.

The more I talked to Everett, the higher I became on this idea of what my artistry and career could be. And the more that happened, the more I *needed* to talk to him.

He sent me digital gifts of movies, documentaries, and records. One day he suggested a writing prompt: "Pretend you are a ghost and you have one last message to communicate to someone you love who is still alive." I wrote three song ideas in fifteen minutes.

Not admitting to an emotional affair when you're in a monogamous relationship is, of course, a form of deception. While Everett had been away for weeks on tour, we'd been communicating nonstop. Then, one night, Everett sent me an address of where to meet him, and I told Eddie I was going to have dinner with a girlfriend. It was the first time I'd lied in clear, plain language, and it tasted terrible in my mouth.

I went to the address, surprised to find myself standing in front of an anonymous warehouse. Everett unlocked it, put his hands on my shoulders, and guided me into the pitch-black room from behind.

"I really hope you're not a serial killer," I said.

"Me, too," he cackled, his smoker's chest rattle making him sound decades older than he was.

His footsteps clacked off in the distance and I heard the sound of a giant switch being pulled. The warehouse flashed to life: a private museum. The walls were painted gold and lined with antique botanical paintings. Giant chandeliers cast pools of gold light into the room and his collection of gemstones and fossils looked as if they were emitting an inner light. Even the taxidermied fox and bobcat in the corner seemed to come alive, their frozen eyes reflecting the golden glow.

Everett walked me to a giant glass display of what looked like hundreds of butterflies, their wings frozen mid-flight. The velvety, delicate wings shimmered with otherworldly colors—iridescent blues, fiery oranges, mustard-seed yellows, ruby reds.

"That one reminds me of you," he said, pointing to one with sapphire-blue wings. "It's the dreamiest one."

He offered to give me the whole butterfly collection, suggesting his assistant could coordinate a delivery to my house. Weeks before, I'd bought Everett's poetry book *Warm-Blooded Heaven*, read it in the park, then threw it out on the way home because I didn't want Eddie to spot it on the bookshelf. There was no way Everett Francis's assistant was going to deliver a collection of rare butterflies to the Pink House.

Everett suggested that my touring with him—either as an opening act or as a member of the band—could be a great way to get to know each other without blowing up our lives.

"Maybe we'll have some superhot late-night affair, sneaking between each other's hotel rooms . . ." he said.

"I'm not really the sneaking-between-hotel-rooms kind of girl," I said. "I'm more of the take-her-home-to-your-parents kind of girl."

"Unfortunately, I'm not the kind of guy with parents to take you home to," Everett said.

When I had first moved to Los Angeles, a famous DJ who had also grown up in Chicago offered me this advice: "Los Angeles is a carnival where everyone is performing all the time. You can go to the carnival. You can have fun at the carnival. But, whatever you do, do not run away with the carnival." I was torn between my desire for a loving, domestic life with Eddie and the desire to follow Everett's carnival wherever it was headed.

When I arrived home, Eddie was asleep with the bedside

light on and an open book on his chest, an attempt to wait up for me. He looked like a defenseless, angelic kid sleeping, and I was nauseous with guilt. I crawled into bed, he kissed my forehead, and we fell asleep. The next morning, I asked for a break from our relationship to consider the questions of *marriage, children, forever.* Our conversation was eerily similar to the *Seinfeld* episode where George tries to break up with his girlfriend but she just keeps denying it, saying, "No, George, we're not breaking up."

"You're my forever girl," Eddie said. "I'll give you some space to think. But our best lives are the ones we're going to live together."

Walking out of the Pink House to sleep on a friend's couch, Eddie entered a chapter of life he called "the Spiritual Sub-Basement," the era when both his domestic and work lives fell apart. At the same time, I stepped up into the most exuberant creative chapter of my life: songs were dropping left and right out of the cosmos, melodies landing on my tongue like snowflakes. I stopped making social plans, wanting to be at the piano bench to catch them all.

Two weeks later, Eddie pleaded with me to get back together. He wrote me a poem with the lines, "My heart is soft soil, yours to dig, yours to work . . . Harvest my heart, drag your fingers through my dirt." He was envious of my new creative fervor, the way I was writing hours and hours a day. "How did you become so confident all of a sudden?" he asked. "What water are you drinking? And how do I find some of it?"

Eddie's loving support had amplified my voice more than anyone else's had. He listened to every version of every demo I wrote and even remembered parts that I'd forgotten, often encouraging me to pull ideas from my musical trash bin to weave into new songs. Yet somehow, Everett's fame and power gave his adoration a bigger effect—I became manic, completely obsessed with my own work and creativity. Song ideas were *everywhere*. Choruses finished themselves every time I sat down at the piano. It was like Everett had cast a spell over me, sharing the musical magic that breathed life into his own songs.

One day, Everett drove his Jaguar to my rehearsal space to jam, wanting to hear all my new work. He praised each piece, offering reflections and ideas. His new song ideas were fragmentary and he struggled to play any of them all the way through. *Maybe love will ruin us / the perfume's sweet as the petals are crushed*, he sang, forgetting the next line. Earlier that month, I'd watched videos of him playing for what looked like a hundred thousand people at Glastonbury Festival, and now he was so close that I could hear the grain of his voice.

At the Pink House one night, nestled under the glow of the projector playing a movie in the living room, Everett and I cuddled on the couch. His fingers traced circles along my neck and face while inky blue rows of light from the screen gave the room an oceanic quality. When I leaned in to kiss him, he didn't kiss me back.

"We have to de-escalate," he said.

"De-escalate?" I asked. "I asked my partner to move out and you want me to de-escalate?" Defensively, he backpedaled.

"We could build something really special together," he said. "I don't want to fuck it up. I want to go as slow as humanly possible with you." We cuddled until five in the morning and then he drove home as the sun rose.

When Eddie asked me, days later, if there was someone else, I denied it, and a murky tar pit of shame grew inside me. I kept accidentally hurting myself—banging my head on a cabinet, stubbing my toe on the coffee table, burning my hand on the oven rack—as though it were subconscious self-punishment.

Everett and I continued talking throughout the summer while he was on the road and Eddie moved into his own apartment after two months sleeping on a friend's couch. In August 2015, Jenny Lewis invited Springtime Carnivore to open a tour. In Bellingham, Washington, in the backstage laundry room, while we steamed our show clothes side by side, she told me she and Johnathan had broken up as well. Jenny and I were both bewildered about reentering the dating pool. I said, "Why is it so easy to make friends and so hard to . . ."

"Make out?" she asked.

"Exactly," I said.

On that tour, since my band and I were traveling in a van, she'd gift us her fancy hotel rooms after their bus left at night. She delivered handpicked natural wine to our dressing room and invited me to sing backups in the choir on "Acid Tongue," a song I'd listened to nonstop when I'd been on tour with The Hush Sound, dreaming of one day going solo like her. I posted videos after shows and Everett often texted to compliment me on how strong and powerful my voice sounded.

Eddie and Everett were both offering me visions of the future. What happened next was like a gambler's worst nightmare:

One second, all the chips were on my side of the table and I was deciding which of these two winning hands to play. Then, boom, all my chips were gone. While in his Spiritual Sub-Basement, Eddie told me that he had gone out with Emily, the actress from his film. He said it was casual, a meeting of the lonely hearts club, two friends nursing their post-breakup sadness. He offered me this ultimatum: "Come back when you're ready to get married. No more runaround."

With two dozen songs written, I was about to start tracking the album with my dream producer Chris Coady, who'd made some of my favorite records with Beach House, TV on the Radio, and the Yeah Yeah Yeahs. A week before I started recording with Chris, Everett invited me to track a song at his studio, Warlock. Everett's name as a producer could have been a golden ticket for my career. The doors of the industry swung wide open for many of the other up-and-coming indie artists he produced. But I didn't trust him to make *my* record. I'd worked my whole career to reach this point of creative freedom, and I couldn't risk letting my record fall prey to Everett's mood swings.

Still—recording one track for fun? That I could do.

We recorded a version of my song "Face in the Moon," and I played his Gretsch hollow-body electric guitar. He took a photo of me and posted it on social media with the caption, "Springtime Carnivore in the studio!!!!!"

As my backing band was packing up after, Everett announced to everyone in the room, "Greta's Record Day 1. See you all tomorrow for Day 2!"

I let out a nervous laugh. He was joking, right?

"There won't be a Day 2," I said to the guys. "But thank you for your work today."

"See you all tomorrow for Day 2 of Greta's record!" Everett announced again, as if he could erase what I'd just said by speaking louder than me.

"No Day 2 tomorrow," I said, "but thanks for everything, guys."

"Sleep on it, Grits," Everett said, as he hugged me goodbye.

The following morning, Everett's day-to-day manager called me to run over the terms of the agreement to have Everett produce my record.

"There's no agreement necessary," I said, explaining that Everett had offered me one free night of recording knowing I was about to start making my record with someone else.

"Sorry to waste your time," his manager said.

An hour after that, my phone rang and I answered. That's when I finally heard it—the bratty part of him I'd known was there, but had never seen firsthand.

"You fucked up, Greta," he yelled. "You had a chance to play in the big leagues and you fucking blew it. I'm gonna keep making fucking Grammy-winning records while your record gathers dust in the ninety-nine-cent bin at Amoeba." I could hear spittle flecking out of his mouth.

"Everett," I said. "I told you from the beginning that I was planning to make my record with—" He cut me off.

"My manager is one of the most powerful people in the industry. You burned your bridge with him and with all of us." I was holding the phone six inches away from my ear and could still hear his whine.

"Enjoy making the most boring record of all time. You fucking blew it. I could destroy you, but I won't waste my time," he said.

When the phone clicked to silence, I felt like I was on an amusement park ride that had crash-landed into the ground. The day before, it was hands-in-the-air, butterflies-in-my-belly, *Everett Francis says I'm the next Joni Mitchell!*—and now, there'd been a dangerous, sudden drop and the feeling of metal screeching on concrete. My words were tangled up in my throat and I couldn't speak. As I choked back tears, the knot in my throat tightened until it felt like a marble was stuck in my windpipe.

After the call, Everett erased the pictures of me that he'd shared on social media. Not only had my chances of collaborating with him or touring with him been sabotaged, but I wondered whether he actually *could* destroy my career if he changed his mind. Would it be as easy for him as deleting those photos?

I desperately wanted two things: to make the record as sublime as it could be, and to win Eddie back. Though I was so sick with heartache that I could barely eat or sleep, I'd mastered the mentality of "the show must go on." I dusted myself off to start recording with Chris. We tracked ten to fourteen hours a day for six weeks, wringing out every atom of creative energy and brain power that I had.

Chris was a brilliant and considerate producer. Each day, he offered ideas and new sonic palettes to experiment with, but never imposed his vision over mine. "The record isn't done until you're happy with it," he assured me. When Prince's estate tried to hire Chris for a mixing job a week into our session, Chris said no because his policy was to never bail on existing commitments. Guitar pedals, which are used to create different effects for guitar sounds, have historically been given super-horny, phallic names like the Swollen Pickle, the Big Muff, the Money Shot. But Chris was so respectful of me and his assistant, Sarah, that when he asked for the distortion pedal, which was named the Super Hard On, he referred to it as "the SHO pedal."

Everett's studio was next door, and each day, my stomach lurched as I watched him pull into the gates in his other car, a black vintage Rolls Royce that looked like a hearse. In what felt like a power play, he hired my backing band for a bunch of sessions, so I watched my friends follow him through the gates into his studio. I was too embarrassed to tell them what had happened between us. Everett's swagger, which I'd once found confident and attractive, now looked predatory and disgusting. He seemed like a vampire, draining life from everyone he touched.

During one recording session, I noticed that Eddie posted a photo of Emily on social media. In it, she was posing in the exact same position as a photo he'd taken of me—sitting above him, her face blocking the sun, an aura of golden light around her. *I'm the forever girl,* I told myself.

The day I finished recording, I walked to Eddie's house and told him that ending our relationship was the biggest mistake I'd ever made. I wanted it all. Marriage. Children. Forever. He'd once said he wanted to get married in Las Vegas by an Elvis impersonator, so I had an overnight bag already packed. "If you want to do it today, right now, I'm ready to go." The look on his face was surprise, then sorrow.

His expression told me what he was going to say even before he took both of my hands in his and said, "Oh, Greta. This doesn't feel the way I thought it would. I . . . I'm falling in love with her."

I was stepping down into my own Spiritual Sub-Basement as Eddie's new relationship cleared him of all anxiety and hypochondria. Now I was the one waking up with panic attacks and searching things like:

27 year old woman heartbreak—death?
Pain in chest—breast cancer?
Die of loneliness possible?

One night, I woke up in the king-size bed we'd shared for five years and reached for him. Finding his side empty, I reached farther, the way an astronaut ejected from a burning mothership might reach for a way home.

I go through life searching
Trying to find the one
I go slip slip
You go slip slip away . . .

I couldn't believe how quickly my life with Eddie and my dreams with Everett both went *slip slip away.*

At the end of that year, my heart was shattered, but I walked away with my favorite record I'd ever made: *Midnight Room.* When Chris invited me in to approve the mixes, we listened to the record front to back. My voice sounded exactly the way I had always wanted it to—powerful, confident, soaring vocal takes with that ache-cry in the high register. I'd shed the imitative layers of vibrato and affectation in my singing voice and uncovered a rawer sound. Chris's production was perfect—subdued synthesizers, driving guitars, perfect 1970s-sounding drums.

You were raised by wolves . . . Can I ever let you in? Can I ever let you close to me?, I had sung to Everett. By the time the song was recorded, the answer was obvious.

You can keep the Polaroids where I am posing nude. Even though I'm leaving, I'll always trust in you, I sang to Eddie.

Unlike the first Springtime Carnivore record, where my voice was hidden under layers of distortion and reverb, the vocals on *Midnight Room* were crystal clear so that every word shone through. Chris and I had focused on the minute details of the recording for so long that it was like holding a magnifying glass over a tiny portion of a grand painting, but we hadn't stepped back to see the whole picture. We'd been nitpicking guitar solos, keyboard tones, and individual vocal takes for weeks. Finally hearing the finished record, I felt like an architect walking through a giant cathedral she had designed. The album was an entire world. Making that record was more about pleasing myself than pleasing my male bandmates or my producers, and finally, it worked—I'd made a record that felt like *me*.

FIVE

NO HOME, NO PART-
NER, NO JOB

SOON, A NEW SISTERHOOD OF CREATIVITY BLOSSOMED IN THE
empty space where my relationship with Eddie had been. Back
in Los Angeles, Jenny Lewis and I entered the discovery chapter of singledom together along with a handful of other newly
single musicians that we knew. The Pink House soon became a
hive of inspiration—jam sessions, backyard bonfires, co-writes,
cooking, confessing. Movie nights with the projector turned my
living room into a makeshift theater, popcorn bowls overflowing in our laps. At song circles, we played works in progress for
each other.

As I met other female songwriters in Los Angeles, I discovered that Everett had used similar lines on many of us, almost
verbatim. Sprawled on blankets in my sun-dappled backyard
while eating a picnic fit for Dionysian goddesses, a few girlfriends and I compared notes on our experiences with him. "He

told me I reminded him of his grandmother," I said. Another friend gasped, "Me, too! He told me that, too!"

It was hard to swallow the fact that I'd acted against my intuition and blown up my relationship for someone who treated me, and all these other women, this way. He hooked us in, demanded our attention, then discarded us the moment he lost interest or the pursuit became difficult. I wondered whether he was playing a game to see how many songs could be written about him.

In my inner circle, I quickly became the most reliable phone-a-friend. Because of a combination of my freelance schedule and my amateur interest in psychology, I found myself fielding queries from friends nearly every day. When one friend learned that her love interest, Tommy, was still dating his ex-girlfriend in another city, she asked for advice.

"If someone told you that you reminded them of Tommy, would you be proud?" I asked.

"Of course not," she said. "He's a wreck."

I said, "So, if someone you loved were dating Tommy, like, if I was dating Tommy, would you feel that I was in good hands?"

"I'd never let that happen to you," she said.

"Then why are you letting it happen to *you*?" I asked.

She groaned and hung up the phone to call him.

Another friend who was a self-described "vaginal hypochondriac" told me she was worried she had a rare STD that doesn't often occur in the United States. "What gave you that idea?" I asked.

"Web MD," she said. "My vagina feels funny."

I said, "Are you by any chance wearing those high-waisted, supertight jeans again?"

My friend went silent. "Only for the last four days," she said, then added, "Coochie cutters be gone!" and changed into a flowy, breathable dress.

I took pride in my ability to help people find their answers, weave their way out of romantic mazes, or compose perfect breakup text messages. Though I could listen endlessly to the dilemmas of my friends, I treated my own pain the way cats give birth—I'd run off under the porch and do it alone, then waltz back in once I felt like myself again. When I was struggling, I journaled, hiked, meditated, wrote music, took a bath. If I was still upset after doing all that, *then* I'd consider calling a friend.

In fall of 2016, Katy Goodman and I launched a nationwide tour to promote my record *Midnight Room*, her new La Sera record, and our collaborative punk covers album *Take It, It's Yours*. The first day of the tour, she told me she was pregnant. "Right now, the baby is the size of a peppercorn," she said, showing me a pregnancy tracking app on her phone. "Soon, it'll be a lemon seed. By the end of the tour, it'll be a blueberry!" She was the first of my inner circle to start a family. I was thrilled for her and also recognized that my dreams of building a family had likely evaporated. I started thinking of myself as a musical lifer, a forever road dog, making album after album, playing tour after tour. I now empathized with my dad's complete devotion to career.

The *Midnight Room* release show was sold out—three hundred people—at the Bootleg Theater. A few girlfriends sang backups, and when we rehearsed "Wires Crossing" backstage, a heartbreak ballad about Eddie, the four of us laughed as we practiced side-stepping dance moves and found harmonies. It was a turning point in my heart's recovery.

After that, Springtime Carnivore sold out small clubs in Chicago and New York, but it soon became clear that I was not a big enough touring act to earn a living. After paying my band and covering hotels and gas, I often came home with nothing in my pocket. I was disappointed that the record I'd been most proud of hadn't broken through to a bigger audience. I hustled, teaching one-on-one music lessons, pitching songs for commercials, and playing piano on other people's studio records, but I was living month to month. Between The Hush Sound, Gold Motel, and Springtime Carnivore, I usually had four hundred thousand to five hundred thousand listeners per month streaming my music, but it never brought in enough royalties to cover my basic expenses. I kept wondering, *In what other business could a person serve that many people and still struggle to make ends meet?*

• • •

In December 2016, Jenny hosted a Los Angeles Christmas for all our musical straggler friends who'd stayed in the city to play holiday shows.

Weeks earlier, we'd spotted Santa suit pajamas on sale at the Glendale Galleria mall, and she rushed over to them with a childlike gleam in her eye and bought a dozen. She fell in love with the puniest Christmas tree on the lot, a stump with the top half of it sliced off, more of a Christmas bush. We crowned a star atop its bald head and strung lights around it.

A dozen friends gathered and we ate tamales and guacamole, sipped tequila over ice, and exchanged gifts. Jenny gifted me a ring engraved with the phrase LOVES WAY, which had been the name of her parents' lounge act during her childhood, and later, a name she chose for her record label. Slipping it onto my ring finger felt like a symbolic gesture of marrying all my friends. Love was braiding itself back into my life.

There was always a moment when our gatherings became a jam session. Katy grabbed the bass and started improvising lyrics:

> *Naughty or nice, naughty or nice,*
> *I've been a bad motherfucker!*
> *Don't buy me any gifts this year!*

This sent us all into fits of laughter, since Katy was one of the kindest people around. Her husband, Todd, started rolling a surfer beat on the drums. I settled behind the keyboard and our friend Kevin Morby picked up a guitar and launched into an off-key guitar riff that sent my keyboard part into hiccups because I was practically crying with laughter. Kevin sang,

> *Naughty or nice, naughty or nice,*
> *I've been a nightmare*
> *A lump of coal would be fair!*

Jenny dashed into the living room to hop on a microphone with our friend Morgan, delivering surfer harmonies in thirds.

Todd escalated the snare beat faster and faster until the song sounded like it was about to careen off a cliff. *Naughty or nice! Naughty or nice!* We all sang, until we couldn't keep up with the speed of it. I'd found my musical family: as part of that gang of Santas, I laughed so hard that my ribs ached.

The next day, hungover, I awoke in my Santa suit and packed my most sensible holiday dresses to meet my dad and stepmom's side of the family for a vacation on the California coast. My brother, my stepsister, and my stepbrother were all happily married with two kids each. I felt like an outsider—the single auntie, the tumbleweed rolling from tour to tour, the only person who didn't have a five- or ten-year plan unfolding as predicted.

On the last day of the trip, my dad asked me to go on a walk with him—just the two of us. During the walk, he cross-examined me about my career plans. I'd hoped my record label would renew my contract, but it hadn't committed yet, so my only concrete next step was continuing to write.

His voice dropped as he asked, "Greta, what's your plan B? You're not going to live in that pink shack forever."

"If I had a plan B, I'd fall back on it," I said. "I'm staying afloat as a musician."

"But how long will that last?" my dad asked. "Look, I believe in you, but earning money is a byproduct of the value you're providing to the world. The more value, the more compensation."

It felt like a gut punch, as though he were saying that I wasn't providing value since I wasn't earning enough for what

I was making. The music industry no longer supported artists at my level.

Till that point, I'd always had an *I'll-show-you* attitude when he doubted me, but driving home later on the 101, staring through the cracked windshield that I'd been saving up to fix, his words replayed in my head over and over. *What's your plan B?* The voice of his doubt became louder than the voice of my excitement.

* * *

In early 2017, my record label did not option my third Springtime Carnivore record, which was a big disappointment. Thankfully, Jenny invited me to play keyboards as an accompanist for her. I journaled my way through the choice: *Is becoming a sideperson a detour or a shortcut?* Learning the catalog of a songwriting hero seemed like it could only help me write better songs, and hanging out with her would boost my spirits. I spent dozens and dozens of hours listening to Jenny's records to meticulously translate those elements—the bass lines, drumbeats, and guitar parts—into intricate piano arrangements.

When we played for thirty-five hundred people as a duo at the Ann Arbor Folk Festival, my voice popped in only for high harmonies on her most popular songs, like "Just One of the Guys" and "The Voyager." A pin-drop silence filled the room while we played, broken by thunderous applause between songs.

During our bows, we both instinctively raised our hands toward each other, a pantomime to mean "Give it up for Jenny!"

and "Give it up for Greta!" but we did it at the exact same time. Seventeen-year-old me would have been floored to see this moment as part of my life. There was such joy and easy camaraderie playing music with women.

My dad drove up from Chicago for the show and beamed with pride afterward. Backstage, he told me, "Being a musical director for other people . . . now *that* could be a stable job. You were the backbone of the whole show!"

Once, when I pointed out to Jenny how she tended to be oblivious to the numerous people flirting with her after shows, she told me that she had a complex left over from when she had been a child actor: She had never gotten to play the Lead Cool Girl who had a romantic interest. She always played the Friend. I assured her that she had officially become the Lead Cool Girl. As a matter of fact, *I* was now the Friend.

I had officially entered my sidekick era. Two years out of my relationship with Eddie, my friendships were thriving, but I longed for partnership again. The problem was that I was allergic to anyone who'd make a great partner. The guy who was a volunteer chef at the Midnight Mission in downtown LA and brought me flowers? No thanks. The one who painted with his own blood? Tell me more! I pursued men who told me in English, a language I speak fluently, that they were not interested in a monogamous relationship with me, yet I persisted, hoping to change their minds by being just a *little* more charming.

On a hike one day, I confided in my friend Jim that I couldn't break the pattern of being attracted to unavailable people. "It's a form of protection," he said. "If someone's not available, you never have to be truly seen. And if you never have to be seen, you never have to be vulnerable. You never have to do the true work of love."

In August 2017, two girlfriends accompanied me on the drive from Los Angeles to begin a tour in Colorado, and we worked in some sightseeing days in Utah on the way. The three of us, all single, read aloud from Don Miguel Ruiz's book *The Mastery of Love*. In it, Ruiz suggests a thought experiment: Imagine that you have a magical kitchen in your home. In this kitchen, you can have any food you want, in any quantity, any time, from any place in the world. You share your food freely. You never worry about starving. If someone knocked at your door with steaming hot pizza and said, "I'll give you this pizza if you let me control your life," the offer would seem insane, because you could make the same pizza, perhaps one that's even better, for yourself. Ruiz writes:

> Now imagine the exact opposite. Several weeks have gone by, and you haven't eaten. You are starving, and you have no money in your pocket to buy food. The person comes with the pizza and says, "Hey, there's food here. You can have this food if you just do what I want you to do." You can smell the food and you are starving. You decide to accept the food and do whatever that person asks of you. You eat some food, and he says, "If you want more, you can have more, but you have to keep doing what I want you to do."

As my girlfriends and I drove through those heart-opening, vast western landscapes, I committed to myself: "I will become a *master of love.* No more desperation. No more starving. No more pursuing unavailable people. I will serve up personal pan pizzas of self-love and compassion every hour, on the hour." Four months earlier, I'd had a wonderful date with a music engineer named Owen when he was visiting Los Angeles for work, and we'd been text-flirting and occasionally talking on the phone since. Our tours were about to intersect in Colorado and I hoped to spend the night together there and ignite the casual courtship into a full-on romance.

In Zion National Park, my friends and I hiked the Emerald Pools trail, threading through the red-rock landscape to shimmering green ponds beneath a waterfall. Afterward, we swam in the Virgin River between two-thousand-foot-high cliffs. The canyon hummed with a potent healing quality that made the sleeping atoms of my being zing their way back into aliveness. Leaving the canyon, I witnessed a newfound brightness on my friends' faces and I knew it mirrored my own. I set a photo from Zion as the screen saver on my phone and computer to remind myself to return to Utah at the next possible chance.

By the time we arrived in Colorado, I was eager to see Owen. I dropped the girls off and texted him to ask where we were meeting. I was dressed up, made up, ready to leave, but he didn't reply. An hour passed. Then another. I tried calling him twice—no answer. By 11 p.m., when I realized he had officially ghosted me, I sobbed in the sterile, empty kitchen of that Airbnb, whimpering, "I thought I was a master of love!"

Conceptually, I knew I was worthy of the kind of love I gave. Yet, I accepted a level of flakiness, lack of presence, and lack of care in romantic courtships that I never would have accepted in a friendship or musical collaboration. Instead of expressing my frustrations, I deleted Owen's phone number and wrote down only the last three digits. If he ever texted again, I could say to myself, *We've got a 207 on our hands*, as though it were a police radio signal in a minor emergency.

I kept telling myself that when I was just a *little* more talented/beautiful/charming/successful, *that* was when I'd find the loving partner who could witness the full spectrum of my emotions and still love me.

．．．

In January 2018, I was driving to Jenny's birthday party when I received a text from Ezra Koenig. Vampire Weekend was looking for a female vocalist and multi-instrumentalist to join the tour, and he asked whether I wanted to audition for the new lineup. A few months later, I walked into their rehearsal space in Glendale, California—a giant, cavernous, air-conditioned soundstage that had six musical stations set up with cables snaking between.

First, we did "Harmony Hall," the joyous single for the new record. I played keyboards and sang the harmonies. I'd practiced that twenty-second harmony chorus part for a total of about ten hours the week before.

"Could you play tambourine with your left hand while you play that keyboard part with your right?" Ezra asked.

"Yes," I said, but swinging the tambourine to one beat and

playing the keyboard to another felt like a drastic version of patting my head and rubbing my stomach at the same time, a kind of coordination I wasn't prepared for.

"I'll have to practice that, but I know I can do it," I said.

Then, we played "This Life," which had a guitar riff that was tricky to play at the same time as singing the vocal harmony, but I'd practiced it for about twenty hours and thought I nailed it.

Next was "Hold You Now," the duet that Danielle Haim performed the lead vocals for on the record. *I know the reason why you think I oughta stay / funny how you're telling me on my wedding day.* I sang in my voice—the melodic swoop between notes, blending the words together, rather than hitting each word individually, the neutral, round Midwestern vowels, the heavy *c* sound on the words *crying, can, carry.*"

"Can you hear how Danielle does that guttural kind of delivery?" Ezra asked, playing the audio through the PA speaker in the room. "Can you sing it just a little bit more like that?" I'd known Danielle for ten years and loved her music, but it felt funny impersonating her voice—like showing up at a party dressed in her clothes. But an audience wouldn't know that. They would just want to hear the song they loved, without being too jarred by the differences in performance. I closed my eyes and imagined Danielle's facial expressions as a way of hitting the notes with her delivery and sang an impression of her vocal styling.

"Thanks so much," the guys said. "We'll be in touch." I kept the Vampire Weekend guitar pick I'd used at rehearsal and slept with it under my pillow for good luck. A few days later, Ezra texted me, "We loved having you in. I think we should go for it!" My best Chicago friend, Samantha, the spunky redhead who'd been at that first song circle back in 2003, was now my roommate in Los Angeles. When I told her the news, she and I leaped around the living room. She jumped up and down screaming, "You're going to headline fucking Lollapalooza!!!"

That May, I learned forty songs so we could play our first show on Father's Day weekend in Ojai, California. I had Vampire Weekend tunnel vision, studying the band's catalog for ten hours a day, all the songs blending into medleys in my sleep. I planned to live cheap and save my salary to fund my next solo record and tours.

The men in Vampire Weekend were respectful, brilliant, and hilarious. The band's *Father of the Bride* record had been completed just before I joined as a touring member. Once we were on the road, we worked our way up to a ninety-six-song catalog and played a different two-and-a-half-hour set every night, creating extended live versions of songs that pushed the boundaries of the recorded material. Keeping that much musical material straight didn't leave much brainpower over to finish my own music. I archived folders of song ideas, short snippets of melody and lyrics, and vowed to work on them once life slowed down.

I loved the job, and playing with the band broadened my sonic palette and strengthened my musical abilities, but I could feel myself being drawn farther and farther away from the more sacred aspects of my own creativity. It was strange to receive so much attention and praise for playing songs I hadn't written. I longed to reconnect to that inner voice, the one that always told me the truth.

By that Madison Square Garden concert in September 2019, I finally had the ninety-six-song catalog on autopilot. I began writing my next record, devoting my days to the routine of songwriting, demoing, and vocal training. I was writing the biggest, most memorable choruses yet. The creative surge was so strong that I could barely sit still—I felt the thrill of pure excitement, my songs picking up more momentum every day. I envisioned that 2020 and 2021 would be the peak expression of my artistic ability. I planned to spend 2020 finishing the record, to track the album the winter of that year, and then release it in 2021. I'd traveled all over the world with Vampire Weekend, playing the most historic stages, feeling hungrier and hungrier to create my own live show, my own next musical evolution.

Then, in January 2020, I first felt that flicker in my voice during the Australian tour where wildfire smoke filled the air. And then we played Okeechobee. And then I got sick.

And ever since that illness, my voice hasn't stopped shaking. I never imagined that the ride to the heights of my touring career would end with me crashing down, sick and silent, isolated in the Pink House.

That pandemic spring of 2020, I tried to keep up the Stardom Bootcamp routine but found it difficult without the ability to sing. I practiced piano and wrote lyrics, though nothing felt potent or inspired. My voice had been my conduit to my subconscious, and without it, it became impossible to decipher the messages of my inner world. I whistled melodies instead of singing but hit an impenetrable wall of writer's block.

During that summer of not being able to sing, I realized that my psyche usually had its own self-regulation process, like an emotional circulation system: feelings rose from the depths to the surface and were alchemized through singing and writing songs. Emotion had a clear path through me, the same way blood and oxygen travel through the body. Without my voice, the whole process ground to a halt and my inner world became clogged with the muck of stagnant, hazy, untranslatable feelings. I was always on the verge of tears but never let myself cry.

In the middle of July 2020, I wrote in my journal: *The world may be in chaos but the one thing keeping me sane is this little pink house. My little sanctuary.* Then, I decided to rent the second bedroom to a friend named Ora. I was excited about the idea of having a new buddy around during that chapter of the pandemic, but the first night sleeping in the house, she broke out in hives and developed a hacking cough, both of which were so bad that she camped in the backyard. She had a compromised immune system that was easily affected by various toxins, and she insisted that the house was contaminated with mold. Ora left after the first night.

Days later, a mold inspector arrived dressed for Chernobyl— double-barrel gas mask, hazmat suit, and combat boots—and

I greeted him dressed for a summer picnic—jean shorts, sandals, T-shirt. After testing the air quality in every room and measuring wall and ceiling moisture with thermal cameras, the inspector made his diagnosis: my house had what the EPA calls "sick building syndrome." The air in my house was thick with toxic particulates.

"If your house was a school, children would not legally be allowed to attend it," he told me. "If your house was a factory, employees would not legally be allowed to work there. You'll have to throw out anything fibrous because mold spores have probably already spread into them."

"Fibrous?" I asked.

"Mattresses, clothing, books, rugs, any furniture with a cloth surface," he said. I looked around. My place was a museum of the wild highs and lows of the previous five years. My closet was filled with show clothes, posters from shows with Jenny Lewis, a stack of Springtime Carnivore T-shirts and merchandise, and my shelves were lined with hundreds of poetry books. The Pink House was where I had written, recorded, and released *Midnight Room*. It was where I had built a new family of friends after my relationship with Eddie had ended. It was where I had started plotting my next solo record, putting the upright piano right next to my bed so I could work on my own songs first thing each morning and last thing each night. And now, the house was poisoning me. *The mold could be the culprit of my shaking voice*, I thought. By leaving it, perhaps my body would recover from the toxic exposure and my voice would return.

"So, you're saying I should throw out pretty much everything?" I asked.

"Unfortunately, yes," he said.

Sanctuary, my ass.

Creative burnout had invaded my inner life in the same insidious way as the mold had invaded the house. For years, my landlords scoffed at requests like fixing roof leaks or broken door locks so it seemed unlikely that they'd spend thousands of dollars to remove the mold. With my physical health and mental well-being on such a delicate precipice, I had no choice but to leave. My journals and my mother's journals were technically fibrous, but there was no way I'd give them up, so I secured them in a weatherproof bin that would travel with me wherever I went.

That night, I crashed with my friend Van. Over Taiwanese takeout, I bemoaned that I had no home, no partner, and no job.

"Greta," he said. "Do you realize how amazing this is?"

Then, with the excitement of someone telling me that my lottery ticket contained the winning number, he repeated my exact words back to me.

"You have no home. You have no partner. You have no job," he said. "You have more freedom right now than most people have in their entire lifetime. You could go *anywhere*." An image of Zion Canyon flashed through my mind.

"I have no job, Van," I said. It still felt like a miracle that Vampire Weekend had offered to pay me and the rest of the touring band for the canceled tours.

"Now you're getting the hang of it," he said, smiling and pointing a finger gun at me.

"Best of all, Van, I have no partner!" I said, now exhilarated.

I pulled up a map on my phone. Zion Canyon was only a six-hour-and-fifty-five-minute drive away.

SIX

THE DESERT CRACKS
YOU OPEN

DRIVING FROM LOS ANGELES TO UTAH'S RED ROCK WILDERNESS, I recalled a conversation I'd had with a costume-shop owner in Joshua Tree a few years earlier. When I asked her about living in the desert, she offered an ominous warning. "The desert cracks you open," she said. "Whatever is just below the surface will rise up and out."

I was ready.

I booked a cheap hotel room for three days, so I could scope out the scene before committing to a monthly rental. It was riveting to be the simplified version of myself, carrying the only possessions I needed to have fun: my Little Martin guitar, hiking boots, keyboard, a handful of books, and speakers. I couldn't leave the journals in a cold, anonymous storage unit in a city prone to wildfires and earthquakes, so the weatherproof box of them jostled on the passenger-side floor. My mom's were leather-bound and the ivory pages had a gold sheen on the edges. Mine were all junk journals made of recycled paper and stuffed with concert tickets, Polaroids, dried flowers, birthday cards, and stapled-in poems.

The Utah landscape reminded me of Mars. Copper-colored mesas, craters, distant swirling gray limestone dunes. Compared with the soft white winters and lush prairie summers of Illinois, this blistered desert terrain felt seductive. The other cars looked like glowing fireballs, glinting in the bright light. The scent of sunbaked clay streamed in through the windows. As I neared the national park, the two-thousand-foot-high burnt-red Navajo Sandstone walls of Zion Canyon stood like frozen flames.

"Good news!" the hotel clerk said. "We have one free bike rental left." As she wheeled the bike out, I saw the bad news: it was a tandem. She said Zion Canyon Scenic Drive is just over seven miles long, an out-and-back road. The park wasn't allowing commuter cars, and the shuttle tickets had sold out weeks ago, so if I wanted to see the whole canyon, biking was the only way. I could either parade my aloneness for the nearly fifteen-mile round trip but see the whole canyon or attempt to trek it on foot on a 102-degree day.

"This will be perfect for us," I said and wheeled the bike away, whispering, *for me and my idiot heart.* As I pedaled in the front seat, the back pedals synchronized in circles with my stride. When I rode past the visitor center, a kid at a picnic table pointed at the empty back saddle with its phantom circling pedals and nudged his mom, saying, "Look! An invisible person!"

That's how it felt being single sometimes. You spent more energy than necessary carrying an invisible person around wherever you went. You hoped that one day the invisible person would be replaced with a brand-new real person. Or maybe you'd still be alone but your life would be so full that it no longer felt like there was a big, gaping emptiness where that person used to be.

In front of a camp store, a group of mountain climbers chowed down on breakfast burritos and gulped coffee. *Lucky bastards*, I thought. I'd been religiously following the acid reflux diet and continued drinking depressing, decaffeinated green tea each day, hoping my vocal issue would resolve. One of the climbers hollered with a Colorado stoner dialect, "Hey! Can I get a *ride*?" emphasizing *ride* as if it were his first double entendre.

Miles later, I was still concocting an imaginary scenario. In my fantasy, I'd go meet Alex Honnold, the world's most famous rock climber who had free soloed El Capitan in 2017. Alex and I would pedal past the climber bros later that day and I'd say, "My apologies, sir, but this seat has been taken."

Entering the canyon felt more like entering a mythical realm than a national park. On the Pa'rus Trail, the desert floor was blanketed with sun-dried grass that was the color of Joni Mitchell's hair. The moonflowers along the trail pulled their fragile, white blossoms inward in the bright sunshine. Heat rose from the asphalt, radiating into my black bike tires. It was so hot that I wondered whether the soles of my sneakers could melt.

I biked slowly, barely faster than walking, while looking up thousands of feet at the canyon walls, which blazed in hypersaturated colors of copper, blood, ochre, sandstone.

Most of my life had involved gazing down—at the phone, at the piano, at the audience. All that gazing down can convince a person that they're in command, the center of the universe. Gazing up felt like a necessary reminder of how comforting it is to be the small one, how riveting to dance with forces far greater than myself.

As if the universe needed to accentuate my aloneness, most couples in the park were wearing matching clothes. Twin backpacks, twin hiking boots, even a couple in twin tracksuits. A family picnicked in front of the Zion Lodge, all wearing matching peach T-shirts. A couple whizzed past me on their tandem bike, flaunting twice the human power and speed. Under my helmet, my face was slathered with so much zinc sunscreen that I looked like a low-rent mime.

Riding through the canyon began to feel like a choreographed dance unfolding as written. The music playing through my headphones synchronized with the external world. Bruce Springsteen crooned "Meet me tonight in Atlantic City" at the exact moment I rode by a man at the shuttle stop wearing an Atlantic City T-shirt. Later, Lucinda Williams sang "Gonna get in my Mercury and drive around the world" right as the sun glinted off the decal on the back of a Mercury pulling into the Zion National Park Lodge. Were coincidences like this always happening and I was usually too busy to notice?

Halfway through Bob Dylan's Witmark Demos collection, the music cut out because I'd lost service. *Silence*, I said to myself. *I can do silence.* Cooling shadows of sweat were already pooling on the shoulders of my shirt as I took my backpack off to stash my phone and headphones.

I was always listening to music, either in the room or in my head, rehearsing new material or chewing on a song in progress. In silence, my other senses became amplified and my awareness of my surroundings heightened.

Like that famous moment in *The Wizard of Oz* when everything turns from black and white into color, there was a richer saturation to everything I looked at. I tuned my ears in to each layer of the soundscape. A fawn broke a branch with its hoof. The river bubbled and popped, moving over stones. The heron's wings *whooooshed* like the shuffling of a deck of cards. I felt drenched with aliveness, as though the livingness of this place were seeping into my body to bring back my own. A whisper of intuition told me that I shouldn't return to Los Angeles, that I should live in wilderness areas as long as I could.

A few miles later, I hopped off the bike and lay on the warm ground below a formation called Weeping Rock. At the top of the rock were lush hanging gardens that seemed to defy the harsh desert environment. Ferns, orchids, piñons, columbines, and junipers thrived in what seemed an impossible landscape because their roots pulled moisture from deep within the sandstone. The prepandemic world felt like a glass that had shattered in zero gravity, all the shards floating in different directions. And my own body felt so foreign with my voice flickering in and out. Gazing at the hanging gardens, I knew that I needed to root down and access a resilience deeper than I'd known, but how?

Once I had been silent for long enough, the voice of my heart spoke up. It said that every time I was *just* about to heal, I broke it open again by pursuing some new ill-fated love story. I'd been in perpetual search of a partner who would love me unconditionally. An older, wiser voice within me asked, *Why can't you love yourself that way right now?* Touché.

It was time to stop looking into other people's eyes to find out who I was. I didn't solve the question of unconditional love that day, but I did know the next step: it was time to go out and buy a bicycle of my very own.

• • •

There's no way I can afford this place, I thought, steering my new bike into the driveway of the Jade Oasis Lodge, a stylish hotel with a clear-blue swimming pool set in front of the dramatic red-rock view of West Temple, the highest peak of Navajo Sandstone in Zion.

When I asked the clerk if the hotel offered a monthly discount, she said they did not. She told me the fee for thirty-one consecutive nights, a number so high that I slipped into a British accent, something I do only when a situation requires an extra level of fanciness. "Thank you for that information!" I said. She squinted at me with a look of recognition. "Is your name Greta, by any chance?" she asked.

I was rarely recognized. Anytime it did happen was usually embarrassing. Once, it happened when I was standing naked in the locker room after a hot yoga class on the verge of fainting.

Another time, I was alone at a diner in Hollywood enjoying a slice of cherry pie at 2 a.m. when a small group of Hush Sound listeners approached me; they gave me the head tilt of pity, and one asked, "Is this what you do for fun, Greta? Eat dessert alone in the middle of the night?"

The lodge receptionist told me that we'd taken a selfie together at Kilby Court in Salt Lake City. She and her husband had bonded over The Hush Sound's music in their early courtship days, and now they lived in the next town with their eight-year-old daughter.

"Do you really want to live here for a month?" she asked. I nodded yes, but told her I couldn't afford it. She went into the back office, dashed off some keyboard typing, made a phone call, and then came back with a discounted rate. I handed her my credit card and she handed me the key to room 404. Having an angel at the concierge desk felt like one more lucky coincidence.

It was heaven in a hotel room: hardwood floors, a kitchenette, a plush bed, Adirondack chairs on the porch overlooking the Virgin River. There was a view of West Temple from my window. Coming here to heal my voice and let my body rest was the kindest thing I'd ever done for myself.

Intuitively, I sensed that a total vocal rest might heal the quiver in my voice, so I messaged my closest friends and family to explain that I'd be available only by email for the next two weeks. I'd never before relieved myself of the responsibility of being a phone-a-friend. I pressed "send" and the two-week silent retreat began.

I biked through the canyon each morning and evening in the cooler hours of the day and spent the searing middays in the hotel room. In the first few months of the pandemic, I'd become so addicted to my cell phone that I bought one of those little timed lockboxes to wean myself off it for a few hours at a time. In my hotel room during the scorching afternoons, I locked the phone away for two hours, then three, then four at a time, rediscovering what it meant to collect my attention, to read without distractions.

After a few days in silence, my thoughts, usually carried away in conversation, began to collect in my mind like water in a reservoir. As I rode through the canyon, I carried a palm-size notepad in the front pocket of a cotton button-down shirt and pulled over every mile to write down scraps of lyrical ideas or other thoughts and questions on my mind.

August 4th—If the body holds what the psyche and the heart can't process, then might my voice be shaking as a psychological reaction to the chaos of this time? A person's voice usually shakes when they're scared. My body, on a deep animal level, is scared. As it should be. The collective chaos, the pandemic, the uncertainty. I have to assume my body is just one piece of the whole.

August 5th—Wish there was a better name for God. The Almighty? Mother Universe? The Supreme Being? All That Is? The desert mystics called God "the friend." That feels closer, as though I could drop by God's house to borrow a few eggs and a cup of sugar.

August 8th—If I want to learn about something, I may as well study its opposite. I can learn the pleasure of music from being in silence, the pleasure of food from being hungry, the beauty of togetherness from being in solitude.

The desert had an extractive quality, drawing up early childhood memories, each one feeling pristine and unearthed for the first time. The crimson freckles sprinkled across my mom's back that I counted during bath time. The way I clung to my dad's shoulders in the swimming pool, the hair on his back reminding me of moss. The time I bit my tongue open as I tumbled to the floor after falling off my brother's bunk bed, then the way I held my tongue in a glass of ice while we watched *The Little Mermaid*. Listening to my parents' wedding song, "Annie's Song" by John Denver, while driving for ice cream one night in Santa Fe. *You fill up my senses like a night in the forest . . .* The way my dad reached behind from the driver's seat to squeeze my foot, then reached over to squeeze Garrett's foot. How, when I was eight, I learned "Auld Lang Syne" in music class, but cried the whole way through because the song was so sad.

After two weeks in silence, I felt unbelievably *free*. My inner voice was coming alive again. It felt like all the scattered pieces of myself—parts that I'd left behind in childhood, on concert stages, in past relationships, in all the cities I'd traveled to— were returning to me. This was the first time I was living slowly enough and felt receptive enough to receive them.

Every few hours of alone time in the park was like taking a

long drink from a cool well, quenching a thirst I hadn't realized I had. I craved more quiet time, more solitude. I fell asleep each night dreaming of the next day's bike ride, the flutter of excitement and anticipation in my body reminding me of the feeling of beginning a new love story. The contrast of light and dark made the park look different every hour, every day. I never saw the same canyon twice.

While biking the park one evening as the sun was setting, I noticed a bike abandoned on the side of the road. It was smaller than mine and strewn half over the shoulder and half in the lane where it could've been hit by an oncoming car. A cell phone rested in the handlebars and the home screen was glowing with a half dozen unread text messages.

"Hello?" I said to the empty field. "Anybody there?" No response. The sun was sinking, and I became increasingly concerned as the light began to fade. Just as I was about to leave to report the bike to a park ranger, a woman with long, dark hair bounded up from the riverbank. She took small, graceful leaps around cacti, choosing each step with the sleek athleticism of a dancer. She had a rugged outdoorsy radiance—wind-weathered and sun-soaked skin and a furrowed brow. Her worn-in safari hat had a leather band around the rim with stones set into it.

As she greeted me, her eyes were a clear, oceanic blue. Her nose tilted slightly downward to a point, like a bird's beak.

"Everything all right?" she asked me.

"I was about to ask you the same question," I said, motioning to the bike.

"A condor was taking flight off the high rim, so I leaped off to go photograph." She said this as though flying off one's bike and leaving thousands of dollars' worth of belongings behind was the only sensible thing to do when a condor takes flight.

She was so obviously able to take care of herself that I felt I needed to validate my concern. "It's just that most people don't leave their phones behind on purpose these days," I said.

She said, "Do you ever get sick of clutching that thing all day? I'm always hoping someone will steal it, but the people who live in this town are too nice." This made me want to be her friend.

I didn't realize how conversation-starved I was until given the opportunity to talk. My voice sputtered back into my throat, as I barreled into run-on questions. *Oh, you're a local? How long have you been here? Do you ever get used to the beauty here? Is there much community in town?*

She'd been there five years. Zion's beauty still brought her to tears. Not much community, mostly just wilderness adventurers and hermit-artists. There weren't many single folks in town, she said, so it's best if you can import a partner.

"I feel a closer kinship with the animals here than the people in town," she said, then pointed down the road. "Look! There are my silver fox friends now." A few four-legged creatures loped across the pavement hundreds of yards away.

"So, you're a photographer?" I asked. She removed her hat to wipe the sweat from her forehead, revealing a widow's peak so prominent and precise that it looked drawn by a calligrapher's pen. She appeared to be a few years older than me.

"I photograph for pleasure," she said. "Professionally, I'm a somatic therapist and a wilderness guide." I vaguely knew somatic therapists studied the way trauma, grief, and stress can manifest in the body as physical symptoms. Meeting someone who might understand what was happening with my voice felt like the ultimate synchronicity of the trip. I was so curious about her. She seemed like an alternate version of myself, living the way I would be living if I'd moved to the desert every time I had wanted to leave Los Angeles. She introduced herself. Sadie Lenhardt.

After that, Sadie and I kept running into each other at dusk in the canyon. Eventually, we exchanged numbers and she offered to show me her favorite trail. Days later, I found myself following Sadie through a grove of cottonwood trees, their fluttering leaves bright as key limes against the soft lavender sunset.

I learned that, in her twenties, Sadie had been an archaeologist and worked at the Juniper Creek archaeological site, which was like the archaeology equivalent of jamming with the Rolling Stones. "How did you go from being an archaeologist to a somatic therapist?" I asked.

"They're similar," she said. "I spent my twenties exploring the layers of the past, and as a therapist, I do excavations on the human psyche." Somatic therapy, she explained, was about helping people unearth their buried longings, fears, and desires. She helped clients pinpoint the physical manifestations of past pain and grief and guided them through ways to release it. She settled cross-legged on the sandstone boulder in the middle of the creek, and I sat opposite her.

"One of my gifts is to help people find their lost art, the art they were meant to bring into the world," she said. I'd never heard someone name their gifts in such a direct way, with neither arrogance nor false modesty. She said *I help people find their lost art* with the same directness as I might say *I was born in Chicago*. Her work emphasized three areas of connection—to the body, to the soul, to the earth. When those things are working in harmony, she said, a person's gifts naturally flow through them.

As I gave her the broad strokes of my life from high school to Vampire Weekend, I spoke in quiet, short phrases to minimize the quiver in my voice. She was an extraordinary listener and mirrored my emotional waves as though the feelings were being initiated from inside herself. When I shared the recent string of misfortunes—losing my voice, my job, my house—her face brightened, as though she knew the answer to a question I hadn't asked yet.

"You've always been a Traveler, but have you ever been a Wanderer before?" Sadie asked. She could tell by the look on my face that I didn't understand the difference. As an archetype, she explained, the Wanderer is someone who has no roots, no social constraints, and has left their usual post in society to look for answers. They don't have a plan but let their intuition guide them. The Wanderer doesn't conform to society, nor rebel against it; the Wanderer observes the system from the outside.

"Leaving Los Angeles to heal your voice in Zion for a month without a plan beyond that? Sounds like a Wanderer to me," she said. I'd always traveled with tour dates, bus routes, flight schedules, and hotel reservations in hand. By her definition, I'd never been a Wanderer before.

Sadie leaned in as if to tell me a secret: "Do you feel like, since you arrived in Zion, things have been lining up for you? Synchronicities, serendipitous events, that kind of thing? Everything going from chaos into alignment?" I nodded yes.

She said, "I call it being *in the magic*. I was in the magic for six months last year. It was the most magnificent and revelatory chapter of my entire life. One day, I slipped out of it and couldn't get back in. If I were you, I'd keep wandering as long as I possibly could. Stay in the magic for as long as it lasts."

Then she leaned closer and her voice dropped to nearly a whisper. "Think about it: Your voice has defined your identity since you were a teenager. You've always shown up as Greta the Singer. Now your body has taken that possibility away. And the pandemic has taken your professional life away. It's time to connect with a deeper sense of yourself than you ever knew was possible, the deeper parts of your identity that aren't tied to any of the things that once defined you. A person goes through liminal passages like this only a few times in their life."

The moonflowers were opening in the milky twilight, their intoxicating aroma, reminiscent of honeysuckle, filling the air.

"You lost your voice?" she said. "I'm so happy for you."

• • •

Days later, Sadie and I sunbathed poolside at the Jade Oasis. I confessed that a singer/songwriter I'd had a crush on had messaged me that day asking me to sing backup vocals on his new record. He sent a demo over, which was brilliant.

I couldn't believe the irony that he finally reached out to collaborate when I can't sing. "He's an actual musical genius. The Brian Wilson of our generation," I said. "His voice sounds like pure alpine water. I wish I could write a song as beautiful as the one he sent today."

Sadie raised an eyebrow. "The way you just called him a genius . . . It makes me wonder if he's a golden shadow."

"A golden shadow?" I echoed, intrigued. She explained that a "golden shadow" is when someone represents an unexplored aspect of your own potential.

"I bet that if you accessed the deeper magic of your own genius, that crush would fade."

Where was Sadie in my twenties, before I met Everett Francis? She could've saved me a bucket of tears.

"That time you were in the magic for six months," I asked Sadie, "how did it start?" She said it had begun after a five-night solo wilderness fast.

"A wilderness fast . . ." I said. "Is that, like, a vision quest?"

"People call it different things, but yes," she said.

When I was nineteen, a Chicago friend went on a vision quest and returned from the trip insisting that we start calling him Thunder Bear. I nearly damaged my corneas from eye-rolling. I knew about Native American vision quests and Aboriginal Australian walkabouts—solitary journeys into the wild world that involved fasting and praying for guidance from spirits and the land itself—but those traditions felt deeply integrated into those particular cultures. Most rootless Americans like me don't have rites of passage woven into our culture that way.

Sadie had studied anthropology in college and said wilderness fasting was a tradition practiced for thousands of years by countless cultures. "Most people in Western civilization are starving for wilderness, and for their own wildness, but they can't pinpoint what's missing," she said.

My whole body tingled with excitement. I felt an inexplicable, undeniable magnetic pull toward doing a trip like this and sensed that it might unlock the deeper psychological layers of what was happening to my voice.

Sadie said, "The simplest way is to spend a few days alone in the wild world asking Mystery: What do you want from me?" *Mystery.* The word practically chimed when she said it. I knew that she meant God, the divine, the animating spark behind all life.

Her last wilderness fast had been a group trip overseen by other guides, and it gave Sadie the confidence to venture out on her own this time. Knowing the Utah canyons well, she had chosen a spot in Bears Ears National Monument. Just as I was revving myself up to ask to join her, she told me that most people spend months preparing—psychologically and physically—for an experience like this, and that three other women from her last trip were going to join her on this one. My heart sank. Of course Sadie wouldn't invite me on such a trip. We barely knew each other.

"Do you ever worry about something going wrong out there in the wilderness?"

Sadie pondered the question for a moment, drinking ice water from her canteen.

"I'm not that afraid of getting hurt. What I'm afraid of is a life half-lived."

Sadie suggested that I try a somatic exploration by asking my body what was happening to my voice and then letting it answer in an art form other than singing. She believed the subconscious mind often speaks more clearly through images, symbols, poetry, and movement.

After she left, I went into my hotel room and pushed the furniture aside to create a dance floor. I put on an instrumental piece by a composer friend that had a hypnotic rhythm. "What is wrong with my voice?" I asked the empty room. I put my hand on my throat. Eyes closed, I saw an image of black tarry scar tissue covering my voice box. I contracted and expanded my back, lifting my arms alongside me like wings. What with the stress of the pandemic, burnout, and the loss of my voice, my body had seemed increasingly alien to me, but after one flicker of a true movement, I felt a newfound connection with my breath, my bones, my blood.

My arms cut the air like a hawk. My heart rate picked up as I twirled and pivoted, allowing each movement to happen through me. "What is wrong with my voice?" I asked again.

My body answered in a startling way: I threw punches to the air. It felt like a land mine detonated deep inside my heart, sending off explosive heat and anger through my chest. My body was angry that I'd treated it like a machine, insisting that it deliver exact results. I also felt deep, deep *anger*. Anger with men who'd hurt me. Anger at my own helplessness.

I danced and threw punches until hot tears were streaming down my face. I was crying, finally, all the stale tears, all the old tears trapped in my throat finally released. My body was covered with sweat, tingling with a new kind of aliveness, my senses keen and awake.

That night, I biked to the Temple of Sinawava, the farthest point in the park, where the road ends at a natural amphitheater and cul-de-sac. The skies had been clear and blue the whole way there, but by the time I was heading back, black thunderclouds had gathered and jagged white-hot lightning flashed every few seconds. Thunder rumbled so loud I could feel it in my chest.

I waited out the storm under an awning at a shuttle stop. With time to kill, I opened a note in my phone and translated the experiences of the day into a poem.

this morning i danced alone in room 404
twirling my joy
like i did as a girl
when he crossed my mind
i threw punches to the air
finally understood how those
Martha Graham dancers
move the way they do
their bodies are bottles of champagne
shaken shaken shaken
ready to explode on New Year's Eve
at the end of an endless year
this afternoon i drank

green tea with honey
the last sip
had those collected little leaves
the one bitter mouthful
made me think of him
this evening
i biked through the canyon
look ma, no hands!
look ma, i can fly!
i mean i can actually fly,
i'm a blue heron now!
i thought of him
swerved across the white line
my wings don't work
when he crosses my mind
he lives in the shadows
but every day
i wake up and
turn my face up to the sun

The storm was escalating and there was no time to edit. Worried that flash floods could make the roads impassable, I took my chances biking back to the hotel. I pounded the pedals as water drenched my clothes. I felt like a madwoman, laughing hysterically, *ha ha ha*, as if the wildness of the storm outside activated some electricity within my body, pedaling and pedaling as the rain pounded on the sage bushes, on the cottonwoods, and that intoxicating smell of petrichor filled the air. *Petrichor*: from the Greek words for *stone* and *blood*. The damp-earth, blood-clay smell of the wet earth settled on my skin, in my hair, in my lungs.

The river flowed with great force, and *ha ha ha* I was laughing hysterically because that bicycle ride was the best rollercoaster I'd ever been on! Because I wrote a poem I might even *like*! I was a bike-riding god, outside of time. I felt like lightning itself.

Days later, I ran into Sadie while she was photographing the gold sunset at the river bend in the park. She was flustered and told me that all three women who were supposed to join her wilderness fast had canceled one by one. She looked at me and said, as she had told me before, "You know, most people spend months preparing for a trip like this. They tie up loose ends, unburden themselves of possessions, work with a guide on the wounds that need attention. People spend months pondering what is ready to die in their current way of living, so that they can create a new way of showing up in the world."

I thought she was implying that it would take me months to prepare for such a trip. Then she said, "But your forced move, this wandering chapter, your voice . . . You have unintentionally done so much of the preparation that people usually do."

"What if you guided me?" I blurted out.

"Would you really do that?" Sadie asked. "Five days alone in the desert?"

"I've fasted before. I know my body can handle it," I said.

"Yes, but you'd have to know the risks of being in a remote canyon. Flash floods, rattlesnakes, lightning, bacteria in the water . . ." The moon was rising, casting a milky glow across the canyon like a vintage gelatin silver print.

It would be a six-hour drive to Blanding, Utah, to begin the trip, she said. "You can teach me what I need to know on the way there," I said, meeting her gaze with an intensity that surprised me. It was hard to tell if accompanying her would be helpful to her or if I would slow her down.

"Are you sure you want to come?" she asked. Could I handle five days alone in the wild, exposed to the elements and the depths of my own mind? I didn't know, but every cell in my body was saying that I needed to try.

For the first time since that song circle when I was fourteen, that twin feeling of fear and desire overtook me. Going on the trip felt as terrifying as passing up the opportunity to go.

"Yes," I said, my skin tingling with excitement.

As soon as I committed to the trip, I dreamed that I was mauled to death by bears. In another nightmare, my intestines leaked out through a gash in my gut. When I told Sadie about the dreams, she said that they were actually a good sign: they meant that I was preparing to let go of my "old ways" of being. "A dream of dismemberment often means the psyche is preparing for a dissolution of the former self," she told me.

I witnessed in her a rare kind of self-possession and clarity about her work in the world. She had a confident, quiet certainty about her therapy practice, her connection with wilderness, her photography.

As preparation, Sadie suggested that I listen to the audiobook of Bill Plotkin's *Soulcraft: Crossing into the Mysteries of Nature and Psyche*. Plotkin is a depth psychologist whose wilderness awakening in the early '80s inspired him to leave his career in academia and create a Westernized framework for wilderness fasting ceremonies. Each piece of information in the book was simultaneously revelatory and also strangely familiar to me, as though I were rediscovering truths I'd already known.

"Adolescence is the stage of life when a person is concerned with social status, material wealth, and social and sexual belonging," he wrote. By that definition, I thought, most Americans never age out of adolescence. He likened that "first personality" to a summerhouse—a carefully constructed worldview, built and adorned through adolescence and young adulthood, that feels like a finished haven. But as soon as that personality is built, that's when it's time to set out into the unknown. Coincidentally, Gold Motel's first record had been called *Summer House*.

He wrote that each of us is born with a seed of unique potential that has been secreted for safekeeping in the center of our being. It is each person's destiny to develop this quality, talent, or gift, and to embody it fully. Adulthood, then, is when a person drops their adolescent ego and offers this gift to their community and the larger world. My sense was that the distinction could be boiled down to this: adolescents ask, "What can I get?"; adults ask, "What am I meant to give?"

When people seek a vision on a wilderness fast, he wrote, they're usually hoping to receive a symbolic mental picture or line of language that represents their "mythopoetic identity," a unique fingerprint of their being beyond everyday personality, social roles, and vocations. The vision that arrives this way is usually a glimpse of how a person is meant to connect with the world. On his first solo wilderness fast, Plotkin received the image of a cocoon and the phrase *cocoon weaver*, which came with the knowledge that his mythopoetic identity was about creating the circumstances for people to experience transformation. Soon, he left academia to build the Animas Valley Institute, which has guided thousands of people on wilderness fasts, helping them cross over the thresholds of their lives.

Our bodies and souls came from nature, he wrote, but our personalities and egos were created in the context of the human-made world, the culture-language-family matrix of society. We must venture beyond our familiar reality if we want to connect with the truest, wildest aspects of our souls.

He clarified the word *soul* this way: "By *soul*, I mean the vital, mysterious, and wild core of our individual selves, an essence unique to each person, qualities found in layers of the self much deeper than our personalities." Lines of poetry by David Whyte were woven into the passage to explain what he meant by *soul*:

> *the one line / already written / inside you*

and

> *that / first bright / and indescribable / wedge*
> *of freedom / in your own heart.*

I desperately wanted to connect to that part of myself again.

• • •

Sadie maneuvered Big Red, her 1994 Ford Bronco XLT with 311,000 miles on it, like a superhero driving a tank. She swerved around boulders and through foot-high creeks as we descended toward the trailhead. When we hit a drop, the sun-bleached animal bones and handfuls of dried sage on her dashboard flew into the air. My stomach lurched up into my throat and escaped as laughter. Off to my right, hawks were circling above an oasis of cottonwood trees. Sadie hollered over the sound of the engine, "If you think this is fun, you should try driving through the Kalahari sometime!"

"You're officially the coolest person I've ever met," I said, having to push to project my voice over the sound of the engine.

"I know you mean that as a compliment," she said, "but I don't want to be cool." She tilted us nearly sideways up the canyon wall, veering around a jagged boulder soaked in motor oil where a less skilled driver must've bottomed out.

"Cool excludes people. Warm invites people in. I'd rather be warm," she said.

"That proves my point. Are you sure Big Red can handle this?" I asked. I felt like I was watching a 150-year-old competing in an Ironman. Cell service had cut out a dozen miles before when we had left the main road. What if we popped a tire, where it was unlikely any other cars would pass us by?

"My whole life, I've been called to the depths of the wild world," Sadie said. She swerved around a second boulder, sharper and more oil-soaked than the last. "And I've always needed a vehicle that can take me there."

She pulled to the edge of a steep ravine, pushing the gearshift into park as a cloud of desert dust rose around us. She rubbed her palm against the dashboard of Big Red as if it were the neck of a stallion that had just carried us across the Great Plains.

"That's why I love my Bronco," she said, which sent me into a tizzy of laughter.

"What's so funny?" she asked.

"You accidentally just wrote the best Ford commercial of all time."

We descended with our packs on our backs in the deepening dusk, the last light of the sunset a pale lilac. Flints of topaz, quartz, rhyolite, and garnet winked under our boots as the moon rose. I was shocked to see anything of value left in the wild world, not yet gathered up to be sold. Then, I heard it, the last sound I ever wanted to hear at that moment: the sizzling hiss of a rattlesnake.

A primal flash of fear shot through me, as though my whole body had been licked by a flame. My breath stopped, every muscle frozen in terror. I could move only my eyes. The snake was barely six feet away, coiled tight on a sandstone throne, head raised, jaws widened, the position of an impending attack.

"Gentle, gentle," Sadie said in a lullaby voice. Was she talking to the snake or to me?

"Just. Keep. Walking," she whispered, and took careful steps forward like a tightrope walker. I followed in her footprints, worried the snake could sense the humid-hot fear in my body. Twenty feet down the trail, when the hiss faded behind us, I finally took a deep inhale.

"Holy mother-fucking shit balls!" I said.

"That was—" Sadie said.

"Terrifying?" I finished her sentence.

"That was *spectacular!*" she said. She spoke in an animated staccato, her eyes lit with a new brightness. "Do you know how rare it is to see a rattlesnake at dusk? They're almost *never* out once the sandstone gets cold. That was our first animal messenger," she said, her voice vibrating in a low hum. Plotkin's book had said that, when entering a wilderness ceremony like this, a person should consider every communication from nature, including animal sightings and changes in weather patterns, as messages.

Sadie said, "We've crossed the threshold. We've entered the sacred. The vigil has officially begun."

If we'd seen a rattlesnake within the first hour, how many other wild creatures were out there in the darkness? This trip suddenly seemed far more dangerous than what I'd imagined it would be. *I signed up for a symbolic death*, I thought to myself.

As we hiked deeper into the canyon and the last remaining light drained from the sky, I started to worry about wild animal encounters, giardia in the creek water, flash floods, and other dangers I hadn't considered. Since we'd entered the canyon, Sadie seemed to be operating entirely in the realm of meaning, myth, story, and psyche, while I was still grounded in the material world where bodies can be easily injured. I was plagued by fears of physical harm and also of the dismantlement of my former identity.

We camped beneath a few juniper trees just off the trail. Damp sage filled the air, the milky moon cast a pearlescent glow, and the creek murmured ten feet away. In my headlamp's circle of light, I emptied the pack of items Sadie had told me to buy—tent, sleeping bag, water filter, iodine pills, a snakebite kit, bear spray, a first aid kit, a camp stove for making tea and coffee, sunscreen, and a tiny shovel, the kind children use for building sandcastles. "What's the shovel for?" I asked. She giggled.

"When was the last time you took a shit in the wild?" she asked. She explained that, in this canyon, we would dig holes eight inches deep, do our business, bury it, and then carry out every trace of soiled paper in a small plastic bag. She warned me to avoid stepping on the cryptobiotic soil—a delicate, biological surface crust formed by algae, cyanobacteria, and fungi over thousands of years. As I knelt to inspect it, I saw tons of pinnacles, ridges, and spires that resembled a miniature city of sandcastles.

She demonstrated her favorite squatting technique. "I call this the Thinker," she said, gazing off pensively into the distance with her chin resting on her closed fist, a perfect parody of Rodin's famous sculpture. I loved how quickly Sadie could move between reveling in sacredness to laughing about shit. The comedic relief made my fears seem less daunting, and I began to feel a greater sense of trust about the trip.

Sadie suggested we write letters to Mystery with all our

questions for the wilderness fast. Before I'd met her, my only friends who spoke openly of their relationship with a higher power were those in Alcoholics Anonymous. Witnessing her eager desire for connection with the divine made me realize how much cynicism I had accumulated during my years in Los Angeles, like salt and rust collecting on a car in winter.

Two voices often warred within me—my inner Believer and my inner Skeptic. Here, in the wild world, my inner Skeptic was out of place. I'd come this far on the trip and I wanted to surrender to the experience. As I reached for my pen, I decided to send my Skeptic on a five-day vacation, promising to renegotiate terms at the trailhead after the trip ended. I turned over on my belly, shone the circle of light from my headlamp on my palmsize notebook, and let my inner Believer fill the first page:

Dear Mystery,
My heart has never been more open . . .

The words flowed freely, questions tumbling out one after another: about how to heal my voice, about what this next stage of womanhood might mean for me, about where and how I was meant to live, about how to heal the woundings from my childhood and from past relationships that still ached.

Two speeds of cricket song filled the air, one with a deep, slow oscillation and one with a *shh-shhh-shhh* staccato. After finishing our letters, Sadie and I whispered our questions and hopes for the fast into the night like children at a slumber party.

Sadie asked, "Have you ever wondered if the Earth dreams

the way we do? What if we're just characters in a dream that the Earth is having?" Exhaustion overtook me before I could answer.

DAY 1

"Look at all these great places to die!" Sadie said the next morning, as she checked out the fasting site I'd chosen. She meant the Death Lodge ceremony, which is a meditation in which the seeker imagines their current self dying in order to invite a new version of themselves to be born. Magnifying our mortality is meant to be an invitation to ask, "How do I wish I had spent my time? Who and what meant the most to me? What did I have to offer that I hadn't yet shared?"

Sadie pointed to a small ditch between the boulder and the creek full of wet, dark red sand and said, "You could totally bury yourself here!" With the excitement of a real estate agent pointing out features in a new home, she walked toward a cluster of baby aspen trees and sighed, "What a lovely place for a funeral pyre."

She asked whether I was ready to begin the solo portion. A cold sweat slicked my back and my palms. I knew she'd be camping just a hundred yards away, but it wasn't the distance from Sadie that frightened me; it was the distance from civilization, the vulnerability of being so many miles from the nearest cell service.

"I'm ready," I said, as though saying it aloud could help convince my body of that fact.

"May this be revelatory for us both," she said. Then she hiked off along the creek and I was alone.

The sun baked the land around me. I handled my domestic duties first—setting up my tent, unpacking my sleeping bag, filtering a quart of creek water and treating it with iodine. I secured my camp stove between a few rocks and set out three kinds of tea: English Breakfast (for breakfast, of course), green tea (a sensible lunch), and African Nectar (dinner and dessert). *What a feast*, I thought. Being alone in a remote place was a rare chance to spend my days naked, so I undressed and hung my clothes from branches of a juniper tree nearby.

Sadie had entered the sacredness of the vigil the previous night when we had encountered the rattlesnake, but this was the moment I entered it: my stomach grumbled, and I knew that it was time for the Thinker. Surrounded by the scat of deer, coyotes, and bears, I dug a hole with my tiny shovel, squatted, and shat the way every other animal does.

Afterward, I spread out a bandanna as a makeshift altar and placed a few stones on it, each one representing a different question. Hours melted away in meditation, but no answers came. By late morning, hunger rumbled in my belly and my heartbeat thudded heavy in my ears. The heat intensified, and I felt lightheaded while gathering water at the creek. Flies buzzed around me, landing on my sweat-slick skin. As I brushed one off my arm, two more landed on my leg. Didn't they know I was here to find *peace*? To find *answers*? They were annoying the shit out of me until I remembered that, if every interaction with nature was meant to be a communication, then perhaps the flies meant that it was time for the Death Lodge.

Under a ponderosa tree, I lay in a cool pool of shade. The needles glinted gold in the sun above me and the sky looked endless. Closing my eyes, I conjured an image of myself as the Los Angeles version I'd been just before leaving the Pink House. I saw myself singing along to Dusty Springfield, belting out high notes in front of the mirror in my bedroom. Then I imagined myself collapsing to the floor, going pale. Now, I would merge with her. Both here in the canyon and dying in my own bedroom, the morbid picture I saw was of my breath slowing to a whisper. I imagined my skin growing cold. Sadness washed over me. If this vision were true, I would never hug my parents again, never hear my nieces laugh, never take a walk with my brother, never cook a meal for friends, never return to my favorite trail in Los Angeles, never sing another song, never sip another cup of tea.

Goodbye to strong coffee and feet in the bare grass. Goodbye, soft linen bathrobe and the taste of a perfect fried egg. Goodbye to kissing and making love and dancing. Goodbye to liquid-gold sunsets. Goodbye to the smell of jasmine when it rains in Los Angeles. Goodbye to riding my bike with my arms in the air. Goodbye to rubbing my feet together like a cricket just before I fall asleep at night. Goodbye to the feeling of a song creating itself through me. Goodbye to heart-pounding workouts, the salt of my sweat, the rush of endorphins. Goodbye to newly washed hair air-drying on a warm night. Goodbye to cold Midwestern lakes and seaweed skimming my ankles.

And goodbye to all the things I would not miss: Goodbye to the jealousy that made my skin burn hot. Goodbye, oil spills. Goodbye, nuclear weapons. Goodbye, mass shootings. Goodbye to that pit in my stomach every time I read the news. Goodbye to paying rent. Goodbye to jet lag and burnout, traffic and taxes, fender benders and jury duty, hangover headaches and period cramps.

As my breath slowed and the visualization of dying became more real, some of these unpleasant things seemed beautiful to me just because they meant I was alive. Faced with the alternative, I longed for the DMV, for the dentist, for the days wallowing in bed with the flu. If my life really were to end today, what would I regret?

The hours spent yearning for the approval of those who didn't offer it. The days, weeks, and months of my precious life spent in the time-suck black hole of online distractions. Scrolling through the curated, digital mirage-lives of other people and measuring my own raw, real life against their manicured ones. The hours wasted in front of the mirror scrutinizing my body. The way my inner critic recited my litany of flaws and shut down my work before I could even finish a thought. The way I prioritized my career over family weddings, births, funerals, celebrations. How many more times would I visit my parents in this lifetime?

The heat pulsed through me as my body merged with the world around me. The wind moved gently through the ponderosa, the same way breath moved in and out of my nose. The creek flowed over the red earth the same way blood flowed through my veins. When a hummingbird dive-bombed into the Indian paintbrush right next to me, the miniature thundering of its wings echoed the flutter of my own heartbeat.

The boundaries between me and the world had become thinner and thinner until they disappeared. I was no longer myself, as I'd always known. I felt outside of time. I fell asleep briefly like this, and when I awoke, I could hear the voices of everything around me.

As a kid, I always heard plants and animals talking, even if their voices were just whispers in my imagination. Waking up, I noticed the ponderosa's peculiar tilt, its trunk angled at forty-five degrees. "Hello, Tilted Tree," I greeted it, feeling silly speaking aloud. Its voice bloomed in my mind, rich and earthy like the forest floor.

"Long time since I saw a human," it said, a playful hint in its tone.

"Why are you at such an odd angle, Tilted Tree?" I asked.

"The water underground runs at an angle," Tilted Tree said. "This may look strange, but it's the only way I can survive. You, too, may have to do some things to heal that other people will find strange."

"Like talking to a ponderosa?" I asked. The whole situation suddenly became so amusing. A gust of wind tickled the pines. The tree laughed in a symphony with the babbling creek and the ravens in the sky. A fly landed on my hand, and this time, when I looked at it, I was shocked to see that it resembled a shimmering, polished jewel. Its red eyes glowed with thousands of lenses. Its vibrating turquoise and green metallic wings looked like they were made of wire and gossamer. The fly darted with such high speed and sharp precision that it almost seemed like stop-motion, splicing through time. It felt like invisible antennae were sprouting out of my body, allowing me to receive more information from my surroundings.

My attention was pulled up to the horizon when I saw a raven launch itself from the cliff's edge, riding the wind's current without a single flap. I wondered whether animals could ever defy their instincts. Humans were masters of it. All around me, every creature was living out its instinctual design.

The sun went down, the heat broke, and gauzy swaths of stars shimmered into view. As I fell asleep on the soft sand after an entire day listening to the world around me, I realized that it *wasn't* madness to hear communications from trees and stones and animals. The madness was my ability to ignore the world around me most of the time.

DAY 2

By morning, I crash-landed back into my body, hunger throbbing through me. Temples pounding, head aching, heartbeat thudding in my ears. Even the bubbling of the creek sounded shrill. I prayed for hours in front of the bandanna altar and no answers came. The only visions that I saw were my memories of the enchiladas from Pasqual's in Santa Fe. That red and green chili! That melted cheese!

English tea for breakfast. Green tea for lunch. I remembered that I had taken these tea bags from a fancy hotel in Paris when

I was on tour with Vampire Weekend. Oh, Paris—those cloud-like beds in five-star hotels, those fancy bathrobes.

Just then, a dog blasted full-speed through my campsite, knocking over my water bottle and camp stove. A woman in her sixties with a Texan-sounding accent yelled, "John Wayne! John Wayne! HEEL!" I covered myself with a towel just as she bounded through the bushes, arriving right at my campsite.

"Oh, hello!" she said, surprised to see me. "You doing the whole Hammond Canyon trail?"

"Hammond Canyon?" I asked.

"You don't know what trail you're on?" she asked, tilting her head sideways.

"My friend brought me here. She called it Mystery Canyon," I said.

"I ain't never heard of no Mystery Canyon," she said. "Where is this, uh, friend of yours now?" she asked. I pointed in Sadie's direction.

"We wanted solitude with the safety of a buddy system," I said.

"I understand that," she said. "John Wayne is my buddy system." Mr. Wayne licked the sweat off my neck and she scolded him for getting fresh with me. Then, fast as they'd arrived, they were off.

The strange magic I'd encountered the first day there had vanished. My journal entries from the day before looked like the frantic scribbles of a lunatic. *The tree said I might also have to do things that look strange in order to heal! I'll find my own tilted way . . .*

My biggest fear before coming here had been the thought

of an animal encounter, but the second day was so painfully boring that I longed to see something wilder than a dog named John Wayne. When my belly pulsed with intense hunger pangs, I bathed in the creek, then lay naked in the shade to cool off. As I was doodling a menu for an imaginary future dinner party I'd planned to host, a tiny black bug flew directly into my eye. I blinked and blinked, a smudge in my vision. I reached for my small camp mirror and held it to my eye where the tiny winged intruder was writhing, flapping its miniature opalescent wings, stuck in my tear duct. I pressed the clean edge of a bandanna into the duct gently till the bug caught onto the fabric and was pulled out. I held the mirror back to my eye to make sure nothing had been left behind.

The tiny mirror, barely two inches wide, reflected only my left eye. My eyes, I'd always thought, were hazel. But here, in the bright gaze of the sun, I saw that my left eye was a vibrant green rimmed with flecks of yellow-gold near the pupil. There were four tiny freckles within the iris, and the ring around the iris glowed a soft, unpolished deep red. Green, red, gold. Had I ever actually seen my eye before this moment?

This single organ was a miracle, the way it translated light and texture into brain waves. The way it allowed me to witness this endless blue sky and the canyon.

Lifting the mirror to my eyebrow, I saw my father's brow, an elongated triangle with a gentle arch. The same brow my niece Gabby had inherited. Next, I held the mirror to my lips, noting the cupid's bow of my mother's smile. I smiled. Whose teeth were these? Not my parents', not quite anyone I knew. Maybe I had the grin of a great-grandmother or great-grandfather whose face had never even been captured in a photograph.

Inch by inch, I explored my body this way. Shoulder, neck, breasts, ears—each detail, viewed through the lens of the small mirror, seemed extraordinary. Every two-by-two-inch frame of my body was a miracle of nature and evolution. There was nothing in each small view that I found a problem with. How had I ever stood before a mirror, wishing my body looked different? All of that was societal, cultural. Here, my body was exactly as it was meant to be. In the canyon, it didn't even matter if my voice trembled, since the sound of it was no better or worse than the warbling songs of birds darting through the trees.

My God, look at this eyeball! I thought, taking one last glance before putting the mirror away. Its inky pupil contracted to a pinpoint. It was a whole galaxy.

That night, I dreamed of a golden mirror hanging on a wall, its surface glowing so that it almost looked like liquid. A group of strangers standing in line in the room looked like a few dozen New Yorkers selected at random from a subway car—people from all walks of life, all shapes and sizes, all strangers to me. Each person walked up to the mirror and saw a reflection of themselves that they hadn't seen before. A frail woman saw herself as a young ballet dancer. A young girl saw herself grown up as a sculptor. A teenage boy saw himself grown up as a father and husband. Everyone looked into the mirror to see an unexplored potential, a hidden talent or strength waiting to be explored, or an aspect of self that had gone dormant through being neglected. In the next dream scene, I *became* the mirror. I was looking out through it at all these different people, reflecting back whatever lay just below the surface of what they usually shared with the world. I felt an overwhelming rush of love as I gazed out at these people.

DAY 3

When I woke up on the third day, I wrote down the dream. What resonated most was the fact that I had spent so much of my life being *seen*, but in this dream, I was the one *seeing*. I felt ecstatic to be a reflector, illuminating these aspects of other people. It seemed that looking through the eyes of love and learning to see people, places, and things as they actually were, rather than what I assumed them to be, would be a crucial step in my evolution, though I didn't know exactly what shape it would take.

By midday, my body felt so light and my mind so bright that I wondered whether I'd ever need to eat again. After two full days without food, I felt like I could eat with my other senses. The smell of sage was feeding me. The sound of the creek was feeding me. The sunshine seeping into my skin was feeding me. I leaned against a boulder and pulled out a palm-size book of Leonard Cohen song lyrics. Every line of his poetry was so potent that I could pick any one and use it as a mantra, repeating it over and over, letting it work on my psyche. *Forget your perfect offering. Forget your perfect offering. Forget your perfect offering. There is a crack in everything. There is a crack in everything. There is a crack in everything.*

I turned the book over and gazed into the black-and-white author's photo. Leonard looked smug. He knew how powerful his words were. *Dammit, Leonard, how do you write like that?*

I leaned the book against the boulder, walked down to the creek, rinsed my body with cool water, and then lay down beneath the Tilted Tree. The sunlight warmed all the soft parts of my body. As my stomach growled, my mind went to Amara Kitchen, my favorite restaurant in Los Angeles. I imagined their almond flour cookies with dark chocolate and sea salt, sweetened with maple syrup. My mouth salivated as I thought of the grainy texture, the marriage of sweet and salty. I got up to pee under the juniper nearby, still dreaming of the cookies, when I heard an unmistakable voice. A voice that sounded like sex and ashes. The voice of Leonard Cohen.

Leonard: Are you really going to make me watch you pee?

The sound was coming from the book jacket. When I picked up the book, Leonard's face had a spark in his eyes.

Greta: Leonard, is that you?
Leonard: When a young woman summons me, I answer.

I felt like Alice in Wonderland. Was this all a hallucination? The wall between reality and fantasy had begun to crack the first day here, but now it had completely crumbled. I reached for my notebook to scribble down everything he said.

Greta: Are you flirting with me? From the afterlife?

Leonard: It's not the "after" life, it's just the other side. This is all happening at once. I'm here to answer your question. So, whenever you're ready to stop fantasizing about those new age health cookies, we can talk.

Greta: Leonard, is God there, where you are? The other side?

Leonard: I've looked for God in monasteries and between women's legs and I've found it in both places. You know why? Because holiness isn't something you go out searching for; it's something you already are. If you want to touch God, touch your own skin. Now, you asked how I write.

Greta: Yes. How *do* you write songs like that?

Leonard: The first step: think like a poem.

Greta: What does that mean?

Leonard: A poem is 95 percent blank space. That's how your mind must be. Mostly blank. Greta, your mind is a hamster wheel. Constant action, going nowhere.

I scribbled shorthand into my notebook. *Cnst Actn. Go Nwhere.*

Greta: What else?

Leonard: Speak like a poem. Speak only the phrases you'd be proud to see attributed to you. Speak less, listen more.

Greta: But how does a person keep a quiet mind when

there are real decisions to be made? Like, where is my home? Where should I live?

Leonard: Put your hand on your heart. Still beating?

Greta: Yes.

Leonard: You're home. You overcomplicate everything. Right now, you could be present in this conversation, but your spirit is off in Los Angeles eating a plateful of health food cookies.

Greta: If you knew these cookies, you'd also be fantasizing about . . .

Greta and Leonard (together): ALL THAT SALTY CHOCOLATE!

Greta: Leonard, when will I be able to sing again?

Leonard: You'll get your voice back when you figure out what to say.

Greta: What do you mean?

Leonard: If you don't figure out what to say, you will never get your voice back.

With that, the book jacket went lifeless.

Greta: Leonard, wait. Leonard!

I picked the book up and rifled through the pages, but it was silent and still. I doused my face with creek water, dizzy from hallucination, and smelled the metallic, bloodlike scent of the cracked clay. The sun slanted a ray of light across my campsite. *Figure out what to say.* I wrote that in my journal. I had dozens of songs stuck in the fumble-mumble stage, awaiting clear lyrics with clear meanings . . . but I sensed Leonard meant something deeper.

As the afternoon faded into evening, I recognized that my body had completely recalibrated to the land. My internal speed now matched the slowness and stillness of the world around me. As the sun went down, a feeling of loving expansiveness overtook me, and my heart seemed to open like a moonflower, radiating love outward.

When I was born, I must've known on some level that my mother wanted me by the way she held me in her arms. That night, I fell asleep feeling held by the canyon with that same feeling. Only once I was in that sphere of belonging did I become aware of how much of my life I've spent living outside of it. The constant striving to prove my worth, the craving for validation, the scramble for status—all of these felt like absurd ambitions and they were all milestones of the human-made world. It was my choice to engage with that culture as much or as little as I wanted.

I wanted this feeling to become the measure of the goodness of my life—I would know I was doing it right when I felt this quality of aliveness, connection, and brightness in my inner world.

DAY 4

The next morning, Sadie burst into my campsite, backpack on, hair windswept and tangled beneath her hat. "We need to get out of here," she gasped. "Don't you smell the smoke?"

I'd been half awake in my sleeping bag, waiting for the sun to rise, but now I realized it was already daytime and a thick curtain of smoke had hidden the sun. At first, the smell seemed like a subtle, distant incense, but once Sadie mentioned it, the scent of fire registered. Sadie broke down my tent while I packed up my tea supplies, the smoke acting as a shot in my arm. With bandannas secured around our mouths to filter out some of the bad air, we trekked back up the trail. The sun glowed a nuclear-orange color behind the thick, gray smoke.

"If we see fire before we reach Big Red," Sadie said, her voice firm, "we drop our packs and run back the opposite way. I think there's a trail exit on the other side of the canyon."

I'd read that this trail was eight miles long. The most I'd ever run was three miles. Running the whole trail on our fourth day of fasting seemed a physical impossibility. Sadie felt lightheaded during the ascent and stopped to catch her breath and refuel with a granola bar. Grappling with symbolic death was a cakewalk compared with the prospect of facing a real wildfire. Nearing the rim, we spotted Big Red. A long exhale escaped my lips, loosening the tension I'd been holding in every muscle of my body. But then, when Sadie turned the key, the engine wouldn't start. She turned the key once more, then again.

"Come on, Big Red," Sadie pleaded, petting the dashboard like a trusty stallion. "Be our knight in shining armor." The engine sputtered to life and Sadie steered us toward the mountaintop. Apocalyptic smoke covered the horizon, obscuring the fire's origin. At a gas station in Blanding, the attendant showed us a live weather map: the smoke had come all the way from California, seven hundred miles away.

I powered up my phone for the first time in four days to read the news. After being in the soft, natural light of the canyon, the screen felt like an assault to my senses. It was so *electric*. I scrolled news of the record-breaking fires in Southern California and read a few articles about how residents were being forced to stay indoors and to avoid breathing the toxic air.

At Mesa Market, a small farm stand that Sadie often visited, we drank coffee with fresh goat milk, a firework of bitterness on my tongue. We ate their long-fermented sourdough bread slathered with butter and honey, each bite an explosion of flavor and a crispy-chewy texture in my mouth. Sadie's family wasn't expecting her back for one more day, so we checked into the Boulder Mountain Inn, halfway back to Zion, to process our trip.

The square room was clean and had a faint smell of disinfectant. We dropped our hefty backpacks on the plush queen beds and I showered. Red-rock clay clung to every crevice of my body, leaving a sepia layer on my skin. I scrubbed and scrubbed. The clay dust was in my hair, under my nails, between my toes, behind my ears, in my belly button, in the crevices of my thighs. Stepping out clean and fresh, I already missed the primal feeling of sleeping on sand.

"Your turn," I said to Sadie, my hair wrapped in a towel, my dewy, moisturized skin a stark contrast to her unshowered state.

"I don't want to wash it off," she said, a lilt of sadness in her voice.

"A little BO won't bother me," I said. She studied her reflection in the mirror, as though taking a mental picture. Then she stepped into the bathroom and ran the water.

Sitting cross-legged, each on our own bed, Sadie outlined how we'd do a two-person "council." The speaker would share the heartfelt emotion, imagination, sensory experiences, dreams, and visions of the trip. The speaker would avoid a prewritten script, allowing herself to be surprised and allowing the meanings to come through in real time. The listener's role would not be to judge or interpret or solve, but rather to amplify the story's meaning and to ask questions that might illuminate deeper layers of the speaker's experience. I'd been so amazed by Sadie's listening abilities during our first few visits in Zion and now I understood that it wasn't a natural gift, but a honed skill.

When I told her about Leonard saying *You'll get your voice back when you figure out what to say*, she said it felt like a koan, the paradoxical riddles used in Zen Buddhism to provoke enlightenment. "A Leonard koan!" I joked.

She said that the dreams, images, and insights that occur during a wilderness fast can live with us for decades, their meaning unfolding over time. She circled back to the image of the golden mirror. "I wonder how your life will change as you become the one seeing and reflecting, rather than the one being seen," she said.

When Sadie and I hugged goodbye in Zion the next day, she knew me better than many people who had known me for years.

Meanwhile, my speaking voice had a new animation, each sentence containing more wonder. I sounded so much more like *myself.* I couldn't wait for my singing voice to heal so that I could sing and write from this place of joy, this ecstatic feeling of my heart brimming over, rather than from the state of heartbreak I'd been trudging through for so long.

SEVEN

USED TO BE A SINGER

HOPING TO CONTINUE THE MAGIC OF ZION, I DECIDED TO LIVE for a month in a hotel near Glacier National Park in Montana. I spent two stunning days exploring old-growth forests and sitting beside shimmering alpine lakes, but on the third morning, I drew the blinds open to see smoke so thick that it blotted out the sun.

Wildfires were now raging in the Pacific Northwest and the smoke had rolled eastward, then stalled against the western slopes of the Rockies. The hotel clerk said the smoke might not clear for a few weeks.

Below, two older couples in tennis outfits sauntered onto the smoke-filled court. "Love-Love," the man in the pink polo mouthed, his serve disappearing into the gray air. A crushing sense of helplessness settled over me. The world was on fire, but most people were maintaining business as usual, oblivious, while it burned.

Having not spoken for a few days, I was shocked by the choppiness of my voice when I called my mom. "I can't breathe inside because of the pandemic and I can't breathe outside because of the smoke," I said, the words strained and tight, as though I had to force them through a barrier to get them out.

My mom begged me to come home and see a doctor. In a rare parental move, she enlisted my dad, who called twenty minutes later and told me about the Finnegan Voice Institute, one of the best vocal facilities in the world. It happened to be twenty minutes from my mom's house and they could fit me in for an appointment the following week.

After two twelve-hour days driving east, I crossed the Illinois border. In Utah, the solitude of the canyon had been liberating, but as I drove through smoke-choked horizons, my aloneness activated a primal fear within me. I ticked off the miles ten at a time, until I merged onto the highways grooved deep in my memory. The 290. I-88. Roosevelt Road. I couldn't wait to see my parents.

In the middle of the night, I parked in my mom's driveway. I dragged my bags up to my childhood bedroom. Purple orchids sat on the bedside table next to a carafe filled with water. I pulled the covers up over my head and slept for fifteen hours.

The shake in my voice didn't have a diagnosis, so I had the luxury of deciding what it was, what it meant, and how I'd heal it. I had a sense of control. I'd expected an easy cure. A few singer friends had had to go on steroids briefly for vocal cord inflammation, and I figured it might require a fix like that. I sensed it was more than just acid reflux, more than just mold poisoning, but I had no physical comparison for this specific sensation. The vocal loss still seemed temporary, and I drove to Finnegan Voice Institute feeling confident that I would be given the solution by the end of my appointment.

In the examination room, I read aloud from a sheet of paper into a microphone. "When the sunli-ight strikes ra-indrops in the air, they a-act as a pri-ism and form a raa-inbow." I tried to smooth out my words, but they caught on every vowel sound, as though an invisible hand were around my throat choking them off.

Dr. Kent Howard, a leading voice disorder specialist, nodded with a look of recognition. He asked me to sing something and I croaked out a wavering verse of "Leaving on a Jet Plane." *Kiss me and smile for me . . .*

"What do you miss about the way your voice sounded before?" Dr. Howard asked.

It felt like a cruel joke, like asking a person what they miss about their house after it burns down. I missed the *whole house*.

"The velvety tone, the expressiveness, the ease," I said.

"Anything else?" he asked.

"The thing I miss most is writing songs with my voice. And singing for pleasure."

What I didn't say was that I missed singing in bed with a partner, singing at bonfires with friends, singing karaoke in Tokyo, writing joke songs with my nieces, singing at band practice, singing along to the radio in the car. I missed leaving funny song voicemails for my friends. I missed "Happy Birthday." I missed the way my body hummed along to the resonance of whatever I sang, how melody floated through my room like a silk scarf on the wind.

After a laryngoscopy in which a camera filmed my vocal cords, Dr. Howard typed AD/SD into the "diagnosis" field on his computer. He pointed at the video on his computer screen and told me the good news: my vocal cords were healthy. Then he told me the bad news.

"What you have is actually a neurological issue called spasmodic dysphonia," he said. The condition results from damage to the basal ganglia, a group of structures in the center of the brain. Normally, vocal cords close between words but with spasmodic dysphonia, the signal between the brain and the vocal cords is disrupted, causing the vocal cords to spasm involuntarily.

"The vocal cords slam shut when you're not asking them to and that's what makes it difficult to hold a steady pitch," he explained.

Never in my life had there been a wider gap between my expectations and reality. I thought he would solve all my problems, but instead, he had diagnosed this horrific condition.

"Spasmodic dysphonia is lifelong . . . there is no cure . . . symptoms typically show up in a person's thirties . . ."

Tears welled up in my eyes but I couldn't make a sound. My mind went fuzzy, and as he continued talking, some of his phrases passed by unheard, while others went off like grenades.

"The condition is flipped on by one of three triggers," he said. "Vocal overuse, psychological stress, or a high fever. Have you experienced any of those, Greta?"

The vocal training with my coach Allie, the stress of the pandemic, the fever in March. I felt like I was trapped a mile underwater and couldn't come up for air. Dr. Howard explained that the only treatment was to inject Botox into the vocal cords to reduce the spasms. He said the Botox shots would require experimentation and flexibility, and that they typically worked better for improving speech than for improving singing.

"If the shots give you access to your high range, then that's when you can sing Dolly Parton songs," he said, "and when you have your low range, you can sing Glen Campbell songs." Dr. Howard must've gone to medical school in Tennessee.

My brain performed an inventory of all the songs I'd released, all the Vampire Weekend songs I'd sung backup vocals on, and all the in-progress songs I'd been demoing for my next solo record, which had choruses that soared high up. Having *some* of my range *sometimes* was not going to work. Most of the songs I'd written require two octaves or more, and the same was true for the Vampire Weekend backups. Surely, the band would have to replace me if I couldn't perform the female backing vocals.

In a hopeful tone, Dr. Howard explained that some patients with this condition were responsive to a treatment other than Botox voice shots.

"Thank God," I said, perking up. "What is it?"

"Alcohol therapy," he said. I couldn't tell if he was joking.

"You mean getting drunk?" I asked. "Does that help people forget they have a lifelong neurological disorder?" He explained that two shots of hard liquor or one to three glasses of wine could act as a muscle relaxer to reduce the spasms in some patients.

"You'll have to experiment to see if you're alcohol responsive," he said. My field of vision looked like a windshield in a thunderstorm.

Dr. Howard walked me into a side office and pressed "play" on a thirty-minute informational video about spasmodic dysphonia, an orientation to my worst nightmare. A half dozen patients with speaking voices more impaired than mine told their stories, and I could hear how the tremor in my voice was beginning to resemble theirs.

On my phone, I searched "professional singers with spasmodic dysphonia" only to find a graveyard's worth of stories about singers forced into early retirement. It felt like a guillotine had severed my old life—one in which I had a perfect health record and knew exactly what my purpose was—from this one—in which I became a person diagnosed with a lifelong neurological condition. I ran my card for $875 and left the office.

When I reached the parking lot, the levee of tears within me broke. I wailed the way children do, my shoulders heaving and shaking. I took a few deep breaths in the car and then called my dad.

"Success?" he asked.

I sniffled back tears. "Dad, I might not get to be a singer anymore." I couldn't even remember the name of the condition, but I explained what Dr. Howard thought it was.

"Oh sweetheart, sweetheart," he said. "This is just the

first opinion. We'll get your voice back. I'll help you get your voice back."

• • •

My mom sat at the kitchen table with the posture of a cheery ballerina, eating her usual breakfast of plain goat milk kefir with blueberries and crushed pecans.

"Success?" she asked, as I walked in after the appointment.

I scanned the medical form to find the name of the condition. It was surreal to read an emotionless retelling:

32-year-old professional singer/songwriter began experiencing "tremble" in the voice after illness in March 2020. Cannot access upper registers. Day to day variability. Patient perception of severity is 7/7. Patient Motivation is 7/7. Adductor spasmodic dysphonia, primarily squeeze-down variant.

"Spahs-mohd-ick diss-phone-eeee-ahhhhh," I read off the medical form and then recapped Dr. Richardson's explanation. My mom swatted the diagnosis away in the air as if it were a pesky fly that shouldn't dare land in our house.

"Every problem has a solution," she said, with her usual unwavering optimism. Spread on the table around her were herbal catalogs and newsletters. BEE POLLEN: NATURE'S ONLY PERFECT FOOD. THE TURMERIC CURE: ANTI-INFLAMMATORY FOR LONGEVITY!

I told her that Dr. Howard said there was a treatment: Botoxing my vocal cords a few times a year for the rest of my life.

"Botox is *botulism*," she said, spitting out the word as though a pincher bug had flown into her mouth. "You can't put *botulism* into your vocal cords!"

"I don't *want* to do it, but—"

She interrupted me, "Look, Greta, you are what you're aware of. If you focus on the diagnosis, your vocal tremor will get worse. If you focus on finding your *perfect healing*, your voice will become steady again." My mom did white-light meditations and healing visualizations every day. She had nicknamed herself the Morgan Horse, since she often worked fourteen hours a day without running out of steam. She hadn't been sick in twenty years and so I usually listened to her health advice, but this glitch in my brain felt beyond my control.

"All the people in the video sounded like me," I said. "Can you just be *with* me in this for a minute?" She hugged me and asked me to write down the name of the condition so that she could research it.

"You can still compose at the piano. I'd love to hear you play," she said. As I walked past the music room, I squared off with the piano as though it were a best-friend-turned-enemy. If I sat down to play, it would reveal once more that the voice I had spent thirty-two years nurturing had evaporated.

In my bedroom, I browsed the spasmodic dysphonia Facebook support group looking for hopeful stories. Over and over, I saw the phrase *used to be a singer*. "I used to love singing with my children," one woman wrote. "I miss singing with my church choir," wrote another. "I used to be a great singer. I'm embarrassed to be suddenly terrible at it," another woman wrote. It felt shocking and unfathomable to imagine describing myself with the words *used to be a singer*.

When my voice had first flickered out in Los Angeles, I sometimes felt a sense of inner brittleness and barrenness, as though my voice were so linked to my femininity, sexuality, and creativity that, without it, those other aspects of myself also disappeared. I didn't entertain that feeling for long because I trusted that my voice would return. Now, at the prospect of potentially not being able to sing again, a desolate feeling spread through me. My voice had been the river nourishing my body, my psyche, my identity. Without it, I worried I'd always feel like a cracked, parched riverbed, the vibrant flow of life replaced by a dry emptiness.

That night, I rewatched the performance of "Other Side of the Boundary" at the Horseshoe Tavern in Toronto that I'd nitpicked years earlier. How could I have ever been critical of a voice that had such strength, such raw power, such texture? I would've done anything to sing with that much ease again, to access even half of the power and range.

Dr. Richardson's words about how vocal overuse can trigger the condition echoed in my mind. When I had felt those tiny flickers of weakness in my voice in Australia, why had I chosen to train *harder*? Looking back on my vocal training felt like watching a car accident in slow motion.

The most heartbreaking part of all was the fact that I'd wanted to sound like someone else ever since that *Like Vines* recording session with The Hush Sound. I'd trained my girl-ish voice to be more powerful, expanding my range and ability and dexterity each year. I'd spent the first part of 2020 in vocal practice impersonating Dusty Springfield and Linda Ronstadt and Diana Ross and Tammi Terrell. When my voice was on a tender brink, an elastic band stretched to its limit, about to snap, I had belted out the songs of my idols. I'd longed for mine to be as powerful, as agile, as expressive, as soulful as theirs. I'd conjured this ideal version of voice, one *just* out of reach, and I imagined that with enough rigorous practice and dedication, that gap would close.

Why didn't I want to *sound like me*? Would I ever have the chance to sing and sound like myself again? The way I'd compared my voice to other people's voices suddenly seemed so dangerous.

The purple orchids on the bedside table held my gaze and a heartbreaking analogy began to form in my mind. An orchid seed was obviously meant to become an orchid, right? But what if the orchid seed wanted to become a redwood tree instead? Say that the orchid seed learns that redwoods grow in high el-evation and drink two thousand gallons of water every day. If the orchid seed planted itself on the high mountain and drank two thousand gallons of water every day while trying to become the redwood tree, what would happen? The orchid would die, becoming neither the orchid nor the redwood tree.

Striving to sing like other people may have contributed to killing off my own voice, the most tender, most original, most orchid-y part of myself.

• • •

I shared my diagnosis with some friends and family, and within days, my inbox flooded with hopeful stories of people who had had to give up the activity they loved most. My stepmom, Shelley, sent me a *Hidden Brain* podcast episode about Maya Shankar, a Juilliard-trained violinist who was forced to give up her musical career because of an injury to a tendon in her left hand. After Maya's injury, she became fascinated with the brain, which led her to get a PhD in cognitive psychology. She went on to serve in the Obama Administration as a senior advisor and chair of the White House Behavioral Science Team. "I've never been happier," Maya said in the interview. "I love using my background to help people's lives." But recapped in twenty-six minutes, the story felt too neat.

Then, a friend showed me the movie *The Rider* about a young rodeo star whose life was upended by a brain injury that prevented him from riding. The director, Chloé Zhao, had met the lead actor, Brady Jandreau, while filming a different movie on the Pine Ridge Indian Reservation and had written the film based on his life. I read online that he'd been cast in a few other movies since and now also ran a family farm. Rodeo-star-turned-actor-farmer. Another logical transition that, even for its improbability, felt to me, in my frenzied state, too tidy.

I also read about Julie Andrews, whose four-octave soprano voice made famous in *The Sound of Music* and *Mary Poppins* disappeared following a vocal surgery in 1997. In a few interviews, she expressed her devastation but also shared that, in the wake of losing her voice, she began writing children's books with her daughter as a way for her creative spirit to reach future generations.

As I consumed these stories about loss and renewal, I wished for glimpses into the private moments of grief and confusion. How did people emotionally survive life-altering, identity-shattering changes? What road map did they use to find their way out of that darkness? The stories made it seem too clean, as though it should be easy to just tear up your old life and collage a beautiful new one. *Ta-da! Abracadabra!*

My heart was so ravaged, torn open, full of uncertainty. Whatever life I'd be living on the other side of this diagnosis felt unimaginably far away. I didn't want reinvention. I wanted my voice back. I wanted the career I'd made endless sacrifices for. I wanted to sing the songs I'd spent sixteen years writing and to discover the ones I hadn't written yet. There was nothing, absolutely nothing, I wanted more than being able to sing again.

The week after the diagnosis, I went downtown to celebrate my dad's birthday. He and Shelley sat on either side of me, holding both my hands, the full force of their love and care directed my way. My dad reminded me of his own story of loss—he'd been a college baseball player dreaming of the big leagues, but an injury had put him on the bench before scouts could see him play. "I never got to find out if I could've gone pro. Now, I've loved my life as a lawyer and couldn't imagine it any other way." His office walls were full of framed photographs of famous baseball players and framed photos of his old team.

"Wasn't touring exhausting?" my stepmom asked. "You

couldn't do that forever. How are you supposed to build a family? A homelife?"

At that moment, I wasn't concerned about the question of touring or exhaustion. I was concerned about the question of *who I'd be* without my voice if it never returned. The writer John Colapinto describes the voice as "the self escaping into the open." Without my voice, it felt like my whole self was disappearing.

"I'll figure it out," I heard myself say. My dad had suggested that I see Dr. Steven J. Frucht, a neurologist who had treated New York Metropolitan Opera singers, for a second opinion. "Second opinion, for sure," I mumbled. "Yeah, maybe touring isn't forever." The words had come out of my mouth, but they were coming out of a body I wasn't inhabiting. I felt like I'd floated out of myself and was watching the scene unfold from the corner of the room.

At dinner, when we sang "Happy Birthday" to my dad, I felt that uncontrollable quiver in my voice. It all felt so cruel and unfair that I wanted to scream, to shatter all the dishes, to set the curtains on fire. But I mouthed the words and smiled and shined my attention and love on my dad.

That night, I woke up gasping from a dream that I'd choked on a peach pit. I fell back asleep and had another nightmare: I was center stage at Carnegie Hall, wearing a silk blue dress, standing in the spotlight. The whole crowd was waiting to hear my song. As I opened my mouth, no words came out.

• • •

Two weeks later, in late October 2020, I went to see Dr. Frucht. I desperately wanted him to tell me it was all in my head. The prospect of a lifelong neurological condition felt daunting compared with something that had a psychological root. If what I was experiencing had an emotional origin, then I figured that it could be hypnotized away, journaled away, therapized away. Had I been unconsciously silencing myself? Had the pain of our collective global upheaval been lodged in my throat? Was it unprocessed grief from the death of loved ones?

"This is my voice—the center of my expression and communication. How could this *not* be psychosomatic?" I asked Dr. Frucht.

But Dr. Frucht confirmed the diagnosis. While stress would amplify the tremor, he explained, it wasn't the root cause. The culprit lay in the limbic system, the brain's emotional control center.

"Imagine your brain is a supercomputer," he said. "All the applications function perfectly except for one: your voice."

"Right," I said. "But how can that *not* be emotional?"

Dr. Frucht cautioned me about the Botox injections. "Singers make their living from a half inch of flesh," he said, and warned me that if the injection was not done with 100 percent accuracy, it could leave me with even less voice than I currently had.

Emotionally, I couldn't wrap my head around a lifelong limitation. I didn't want to accept the diagnosis. I maintained a healthy skepticism when Western doctors diagnosed "forever" conditions because I wanted to believe in my body's capacity for miraculous healing. Spooked by the needle-through-the-neck injection and resistant to signing up for an expensive procedure three to four times a year, I decided to address the Physical, Intellectual, Emotional, and Spiritual aspects of healing first—my PIES. I needed to heal my damn PIES. Physically, I'd pushed my voice and body to burnout and needed to rest. Intellectually, I wanted to study the brain and nervous system to better understand what was happening inside me. Emotionally, I'd been so overwhelmed with fear and uncertainty that I felt like I had an anvil on my chest every time I tried to take a deep breath. Without my voice, I couldn't be creative or work, so I needed to prioritize healing like it was a full-time job.

People who are desperate for a cure will try anything. I opened myself to the full spectrum of healing techniques, everything from having my fifth chakra cleansed by an energy healer to signing up for weekly speech therapy with a traditional ENT. I began an exploration of healing modalities including eye movement desensitization and reprocessing (EMDR) therapy, acupuncture, new varieties of mindfulness meditation, microdosing psilocybin (aka magic mushrooms), electrostimulation therapy, toning my vagus nerve, shamanic journeying, Emotional Freedom Technique, prayer, and more cleanses than Gwyneth Paltrow.

Packages started arriving at my mom's house. I came down to the kitchen one morning to see the supplies she had gathered for my *miraculous healing*—a chalky and bitter mold cleanse powder that I would drink three times a day to draw any remaining toxic particulates out of my body. She'd bought a handful of books by the Medical Medium, a self-proclaimed medium who says that he receives healing information from a spirit. One woman on the spasmodic dysphonia Facebook group said that the Medical Medium diet had healed her SD.

My mom said, "You know about leaky gut, right?" She was decades ahead of the mainstream when it came to understanding that the gut is the "second brain" of the body, translating digestion into emotional experience and hormonal states.

"Yes, I know about leaky gut," I said.

Then, like a scientist finally reaching a eureka moment, she said, "Now doctors think there's also leaky throat and leaky brain!"

"So, am I supposed to call a doctor or hire a plumber?" I said.

She didn't laugh. She'd been researching my condition like a PhD student and was determined to heal me with juice, herbs, and motherly love.

"We'll begin each day with thirty-two ounces of lemon water upon rising, followed by thirty-two ounces of fresh-made celery juice, plus a few 'brain shots' throughout the day to draw toxins out of the body," she said, reciting the Medical Medium's protocol. Being proactive and having a plan gave me a sense of control.

We drank our lemon juice and then waited fifteen minutes. We made our celery juice, poured it into wine glasses, and then clinked our glasses together. "To getting your voice back," she said.

"To getting my voice back," I said, and smiled.

My mom had invested so much energy, time, and money into healing me that I wanted to be a grateful and willing participant. Greta Sunshine was ready to sing again. Greta Sunshine loved white-light meditations. Greta Sunshine was ready to say *Abracadabra!*

Privately, I swung like a pendulum between hope and despair. One minute, I'd be fiercely determined to heal; the next, paralyzed by the terror of never recovering. As I pushed my grief deeper down, the nightmares worsened. A few days after we began the healing regimen, I dreamed I was boarding a flight at LAX and when the desk clerk asked for my ID, my photograph had disappeared from my passport. When the clerk offered to fingerprint me instead, I held up my hands and realized that even my fingerprints were gone.

That week, I began seeing Lori Sonnenberg, a speech therapist who had a warm smile and a voice with perfectly balanced Mary Poppins–esque diction (Julie Andrews would have approved). In our first session, she taught me speech workarounds, such as an airflow technique in which I imagined "skating" words out on flows of breath. From her little Zoom square on the computer screen, she demonstrated the method.

"Whhhhhhheelbarrow," Lori spoke-sang, emphasizing the *wh* sound with a gust of air behind it and letting the rest of the word float out.

"Wheeeeelbarrow," I imitated, with the breathiness of a ghost haunting a medieval castle.

"Whhhhhhhhhhhhhere is the whhhhheeeeelbarrow?" she asked.

"Whhhhhhhhhhhhhere is the wheelbarrow?" I imitated. Apparently I was the ghost of the gardener in this medieval castle.

"Whhhhhhhhhhhhhhy me?" she demonstrated next.

"Do you really make your SD patients ask 'Why me?'" I asked.

"Oh, gosh, gosh, I was just thinking of *wh* phrases," she said, blushing. "But you probably are thinking *Why me?*, right?"

I'd read that spasmodic dysphonia affects two out of every one hundred thousand people. Yes, *Why the hell me?*

"How do people emotionally survive this?" I said. "How does a singer live with a broken voice?"

"It's not a broken voice," she corrected me. "It's just a *different* voice."

I didn't want a *different* voice. I wanted *my* voice.

"For now," she said, "the best thing is to stop comparing your current voice to the one you used to have. If we start exactly where we are, then we can celebrate every improvement as a win."

In the following weeks, I learned that Brian Littrell of the Backstreet Boys also had a form of dysphonia, and that he had found success with Botox treatments. I watched dozens of "before and after" videos—he performed again, but with a changed voice.

I also learned that Shania Twain had lost her voice for seven years because of nerve damage from Lyme disease, but she recovered it after a successful surgery that reconnected different vocal cord nerves. She technically had muscle tension dysphonia, the sister condition to mine. Watching her postsurgery performances, I recognized the speech therapy techniques I was learning—the way she now "punched" consonants, the way she skated the words out on the flows of air. These stories offered some hope. But I sensed that, even if I regained some semblance of my old voice, it might never be the same as it had been.

I dug out a bottle of natural red wine from the dusty alcohol cabinet downstairs, uncorked it, and drank a glass, then another. Wine was not on the cleanse program, but I needed to see whether I was "alcohol responsive." I'd mostly stopped drinking in my thirties when the hangovers no longer felt worth the joy of the buzz.

Warmth spread through my body with each sip. Tension released from my shoulders first, then from my jaw, then from my throat. *No wonder people do this*, I thought. *What was I even worried about? Pandemic schmandemic!*

When my body felt like a lava lamp, I sat behind my keyboard and sang that unfinished song I'd been working on. *Woke up in a cold sweat from a dream I don't understand yet . . .*

When I heard the melody in my mind, it seemed so clear and easy, but when I tried to sing, my voice was uncontrollable. The sound of my voice was still gravelly and I couldn't hold a steady pitch, so I drank another two glasses of wine.

Out of nowhere, Cher infiltrated my brain and began singing *Do you believe in life after love?* I tried to sing along but couldn't hold the pitches. Then the song "Sweet Caroline" came into my mind. It was like a jukebox had exploded in my brain. *Pull yourself together*, I thought, but I was so sloppy that nothing made sense. I kept singing the kinds of choruses you hear on dance floors at bat mitzvahs. *Oooo, I wanna dance with somebody! I wanna feel the heat with somebody! I wanna write a chorus like that*, I thought. *Up all night to get lucky!* One massive chorus after another, I kept singing with a slurring, tone-deaf, off-key voice.

When I went back to my song and tried to belt the high notes, my voice was all screech and strain with no tone. The next morning, I woke up with a piercing headache and a sluggish body, no closer to recovering my voice.

Once I was on the wavelength of loss, I couldn't stop looking back at other painful experiences—the deaths of loved ones, the heartbreaks, the breakups, the existential aches. Beyond my own life, I grieved the ecological destruction, the inflamed hatred and worsening division as we neared the presidential election, the uncertainty of the pandemic. The writer adrienne maree brown described the emotional tenor of that season of the pandemic this way: "Everyone needs more than anyone can give."

"The Green Ribbon," a quirky horror story I loved as a child, circled repeatedly in my mind. It was about a girl who always wore a green ribbon around her neck. When she grew up and her husband eventually removed the ribbon, her head fell off. The ribbon wasn't just a superficial adornment—it had been the only thing keeping her alive. If I couldn't recover my voice, I worried my whole life would unravel.

When I was sick of stewing in self-pity and needed to get out of the house, I set off for long, aimless drives until the density of suburban chain malls and neighborhoods became sparser and the skyline was just farmland. Why do people call it a *joyride*? What I was doing each night was obviously a depression ride. I coasted the quiet roads, blasting records to drown out the thrashing of my own thoughts. My mom and dad loved me and they were supporting me in the ways they could, but I felt deeply isolated by the fact that they'd never be able to truly understand what I was going through.

My mom's rose-colored view of the world and relentless optimism sometimes meant that darker emotions didn't even register for her. My dad was so practical that his way of helping was to research and enact various fix-it methods. Find the right doctors. Try the right treatments. I recalled our conversation from years ago when he suggested a plan B career. He may have been right.

One night, a harvest moon was rising at the end of a farm road. It looked like a golden egg yolk floating over the horizon. I wanted to drive right into the moon and out of this existence, to disappear completely. The weight of living felt unbearable. It was like an implosion of despair had gone off inside of me. *If I self-destructed now*, I thought, *everyone would understand.* A morbid thought flashed through my mind: *What if there was a way to fall asleep tonight and just not wake up tomorrow?* But then I imagined my mom finding me, calling my dad . . . and a wave of nausea overtook me.

I ended up in Sugar Grove, Illinois, more than an hour from my house. On the way back, I stopped in Glen Ellyn, the town where Eileen had lived when we were teenagers. I drove down the quiet suburban streets until I arrived at her old house. A light was glowing in her old bedroom window. Someone else's posters were hanging on the wall. Someone else was probably winding down, about to fall asleep in that room.

Nothing good ever stays in my life. I've always tried to stay strong on my own but I can't do it anymore.

When I'd first read her suicide note, I'd wondered: *How could she have been so low that her life no longer seemed worth living?* But now that I was processing my own heavy, pervasive loss, I understood how it could spread outward like an oil spill, staining everything it touched.

Out of nowhere, a line of the poet Rilke appeared in my mind: *No feeling is final.*

Gazing at Eileen's old room, I knew that I was going to live one hour at a time. I was going to take deep breaths until my breathing diffused the suffocating feelings of despair. I put all my faith in one line of poetry. I would keep breathing and I would wait for the feeling to change.

• • •

"Mom, I'm so depressed that it kind of scares me," I said at breakfast the next morning. Though my body felt healthier from the cleanse, my voice hadn't improved.

"Maybe we should do a bowel cleanse," she suggested, and started rifling through her herbal cabinet.

"I think it's more than my gut," I said.

"You've barely even touched the piano," she said. "The house is so quiet."

"Music just doesn't feel fun right now," I said. Her face looked as though I'd just announced it was time for her to go murder a Labrador puppy with me.

I stepped outside onto the porch. The warmth on my skin felt like a glimpse of physical pleasure. I remembered how warm the sun had felt in Zion, how the sandstone radiated with it. The light was so bright that I could've set the dry grass on fire by turning my bike mirror at the wrong angle. The sun on my face felt almost like physical tenderness, the loving touch of a partner. I felt so far away from having that again.

As though my mom could read my mind, she asked through the screen door, "Would Eddie ever take you back?"

"I don't think so, Mom."

"How could he *possibly* be happy with the actress?" My mom never referred to Eddie's partner by her actual name.

"He's been in that relationship as long as we were together," I said. "I think he's really happy, Mom."

I realized how stale my bedroom felt only upon reentering it after being in the fresh air. The room looked like a cliché rom-com setting of a recently divorced dad: dirty dishes on the bedside table, a chocolate bar wrapper on the floor, an empty wine bottle from last night's alcohol therapy, a bottle of oil for masturbating.

I used to be able to draw on dozens of sexual fantasies, but now all I could fantasize about was being held, leaning my head on the chest of a strong and steady partner, having my hair tucked behind my ears. I fantasized about drinking coffee in bed and reading aloud to a partner and holding hands while falling asleep.

On the phone, I told Sadie how lost I felt. "Being lost is the Wanderer's journey," she said. "If you weren't lost, you wouldn't be changing." But I didn't feel like I was on a Wanderer's journey anymore. I felt like Icarus, burned to a crisp after flying too close to the sun. Or like Amelia Earhart, journey over, body never found.

"When was the last time you felt even the tiniest spark of magic?" Sadie asked. I rewound my memory. *Escalante.*

When we had driven through Escalante, Utah, on the way back to Zion after the wilderness fast, I had lit up with that whole-body, balloon-floating-out-of-my-chest kind of hope. Sadie suggested that I should go there.

I couldn't tell which was crazier: moving to a place two-thousand miles away where I knew no one because I had once felt a tiny glimmer of possibility there, or sleeping in my childhood bed and pretending to be Greta Sunshine for the rest of the pandemic.

I scrolled rental listings while we talked. The first house that came up was called *La Luna.* The moon. The house was at the edge of town closest to the Grand Staircase monument, a natural preserve full of slot canyons, waterfalls, and countless hiking trails. The town would be quiet. The sunshine would be bright. *Escalante.* I liked how the word rolled across my tongue. I looked up the meaning: *the staircase.* I'd hit my rock bottom, and I was ready to take the first steps back up.

EIGHT

TURN THAT ACHE INTO AN OFFERING

ROLLING INTO ESCALANTE, UTAH, POPULATION 809, I SAW three establishments on the main drag that were open in the off-season: the US post office, Griffin Grocery, and Nemo's burgers. Beneath the faded awning of Nemo's was an eight-foot-tall plywood cutout of Big Foot with a painted message that read, "Be like Bigfoot: Social Distancing World Champion!" Then, twenty steps farther down Main Street, I saw a handwritten poem on the community chalkboard which suggested that COVID was a hoax, that masks are no good, and that "those scientists' heads are all made of wood."

Driving the dusty road a few blocks from Main Street to my rental house, a shiver of fear ran through me as I saw Confederate flags hanging from two homes and a Trump flag, large enough that a class of kindergartners could use it as a parachute, waving in a front lawn. Next up, a house with Tibetan prayer flags and another house with a Toyota Prius in the driveway that had a "COEXIST" bumper sticker.

The listing for La Luna hadn't conveyed how jarringly out of place the house would feel on this street. Nestled among muted 1970s ranch houses, La Luna was a vibrant yellow rectangle, a futuristic art house defying the neighborhood's conservative aesthetic—as if Ziggy Stardust had showed up to a Sunday church service.

One entire wall of the house was a window through which I could see a vast view of the Grand Staircase formation. Bathed in the golden light of the setting sun, the rock formation resembled a giant, unrolled scroll, different shades of sandstone, ochre, and rust at each wave. The distinct geologic layers reminded me of the sand bottle art I used to make as a kid. Cows grazed in a wide-open pasture between me and the Grand Staircase, oblivious to the geological marvel behind them. The sunset was cherry blossom pink, the clouds so billowy and soft that I imagined they'd taste like a meringue. I brought my speakers in from the car and set them up first. Ambient and classical music only this month—no voices, I'd decided.

That first night there, I invented a stargazing routine to stay warm in desert winter temperatures:

Step 1: Dress in thermal long johns.
Step 2: Dance or do calisthenics in the living room to raise my core temperature.
Step 3: Zip into my 0-degree thermal sleeping bag, sealing my body heat into the bag with me.

Step 4: Bunny-hop out the door onto the porch and recline on the lawn chair.

Step 5: STARGAZE. Enjoy feeling like a hot potato wrapped in foil.

In this region of Utah, thousands of stars are visible on a clear night. It may as well be millions. The starlight was so bright and the night air so cold that it felt like drinking a black pearlescent wine.

A wave of relief came over me: I didn't have to pretend to be Greta Sunshine anymore. I didn't have to be charming. I didn't have to be *anything*. I just had to *be*. Picking up and traveling to live in solitude in a place of wild beauty was a remarkable privilege, one that wasn't available to most people with families, homes, community roots, and responsibilities. Even though the choice to go to Escalante had arisen from great pain and uncertainty in my life, I still recognized my time there as a precious gift. Vampire Weekend had continued to support me financially, providing the rare freedom for an opportunity like this.

There, under the stars, I could shed any masks that I'd worn. Who was I when no one was reinforcing the current version of my identity? Emotionally attuning to other people was a skill that allowed me to thrive in friendships and in bands, but sometimes it meant that I let other people's desires and emotions take precedence over my own. Being alone meant I didn't have to perform cheerfulness for my mom or focus on solutions for my dad or update all my friends on what was happening and how I felt about it.

Under the stars that first night, I recognized that there were two possible kinds of healing. Maybe I *would* experience a literal healing of my voice and be able to sing again. If that were the case, I'd go on with my artistic life as planned. If my voice *couldn't* heal, though, I'd have to figure out how to heal my spirit.

In a newsletter that had arrived earlier that week, the writer Sophie Strand shared something her friend Mary Evelyn Pritchard had told her: "Health is the amount of joy in a person's life. Even a person with chronic illness can aspire to that." But how would I find my joy if singing were no longer possible?

The soundscape was devoid of any human-made sounds. There was only a whisper of windblown sand, a rustle of creosote bushes. I could hear the blood moving in my ears, a subtle, airy churn, as though I were listening to conch shells. The silence had a gravitational pull, a romantic quality. The night air bit at my cheeks and eyes, and when my hot potato temperature cooled to soggy French fry territory, I bunny-hopped inside and fell asleep. The cry of coyotes woke me around 3 a.m. and I looked out the window to see two dogs next door cuddle beneath a heat lamp in a doghouse, surrounded by a dust of freshly fallen snow. *Lucky pups.* I brushed my hand against my cheek, tucked the hair behind my ears, and put myself back to bed.

· · ·

Frozen with writer's block since my diagnosis, I signed up for a songwriting workshop about creative bravery with Mary

Gauthier. I had discovered Mary's work seven years before, when I heard her say this in an interview: "If my voice isn't shaking the first time I play a new song live, I'm not being honest enough." I immediately read every lyric she'd ever written.

Mary's songs are full of longing, lost characters—orphans, wanderers who can't find homes, veterans who can't end the war in their heads. Her records are raw and unflinching accounts about her struggles with addiction, coming to terms with her sexuality, and the abandonment wounds of being given up for adoption. Mary couldn't even speak her dream of being a song- writer until she was thirty-two, when a DUI prompted her entry into rehab. Finally clearheaded, she sat in the group therapy cir- cle and named her deepest and most terrifying desire: *I want to be a songwriter*, she said. She had never even held a guitar.

In the thirty years since that time, she's released stunning folk records that have been nominated for Grammys and have topped the Americana charts. Her songs have been recorded by Dolly Parton and Jimmy Buffett.

Even if I couldn't sing, I could try writing song lyrics. If anyone could turn me into a lyricist again, it would be her.

On a cold, clear Sunday morning, I settled myself at the ta- ble and logged into the class. Mary welcomed everyone. She had short, silver hair, and when her eyes crinkled up in a smile, she seemed far younger than her fifty-nine years. She wore a button- down shirt with a vest over it, classic troubadour attire. Her part- ner in life and music, Jaimee Harris, sat beside her in the home where they lived together. Behind them, a rainbow American flag hung from the wall above a shelf of books and records.

"If you're not afraid when you play a song live for the first time, you're either insane or you're not saying anything meaningful," she said, echoing the statement that made me fall in love with her work in the first place. "If we want to write brave songs, it is necessary to trigger our fear." Back in our hunter-gatherer days, she explained, if we did anything to alienate ourselves from our social group, it meant death. These days, if we get rejected by the group, we won't die, but the animal part of our brain still thinks we might.

Rejection was everywhere, she said, especially in the age of anonymous internet haters. So we needed to prepare ourselves to make and share brave art, knowing that it would definitely be rejected, at least by some. Once, when she posted a photo of herself with a baby, the daughter of two of her Canadian fans, a commenter wrote, "What's the big deal about babies? I don't like babies." Mary said, "If there's a baby-hating contingent out there, you can trust that, no matter what you share, there will *always* be someone whose knee-jerk reaction is to hate it."

"So," Mary said, "what's on the all-you-can-eat buffet of terror today? What fears keep you from writing and sharing brave songs?" People unmuted themselves to speak: One man felt he should be better after forty years of writing. Another said he was afraid of hurting his parents by naming the painful aspects of his childhood. A woman confessed she was worried that if she actually started writing, she may be forced to realize she is not the secret genius she has always imagined herself to be.

"Who the hell do I think I am to devote this much time to making my own art?" one person said. "Who the hell am I to spend so much time expressing myself and hoping other people will listen?"

Mary's answer: "You are a humble servant to truth and beauty. It's the same answer every time." I loved that idea, as though I were just placing my tiny, glowing candle on the altar of all the songs that had ever existed.

Mary suggested that as fears arose within us during the following week, we should write them down and then respond to them from the wiser part of ourselves. When I signed off from the first class, I still would've rather cleaned my shower with a toothbrush than write a song, but I felt more *open* to the idea.

The next day, I decided to try Mary's exercise by writing down my fears and entering into conversation with them.

Fear: I'll never write a great song again without my voice.

Answer to Fear: How do you know if you don't try?

Fear: I'm afraid my voice will never return.

Answer to Fear: If it doesn't, you'll have to find another way to express yourself. Maybe you'll learn how to paint or how to cook. You will find another outlet.

Fear: I'm afraid I'll go broke. I can't earn money without my voice. I have no higher education and no backup plan.

Answer to Fear: You've never *tried*. How do you know until you try?

Fear: What if this is the beginning of something worse? Multiple sclerosis. Parkinson's. Some neurological issue that will progress quickly.

Answer to Fear: Your neurologist ruled all that out. For now, trust him. And if this were the beginning of something worse, that could be an incentive to live as fully as possible right now.

Fear: I'm afraid that losing my voice will force me into a state of total social isolation. I'll become depressed. And I'll never date again because conversation will be too challenging.

Answer to Fear: Oh, sweetie pie, who decided to spend forty days alone in the desert?

I filled pages and pages like this. I wondered how I'd been able to go to the grocery store or brush my teeth while carrying around that much fear. The more I wrote, the more I realized that fear wasn't me: fear was a parasite clinging to me for survival, a leech sucking the life from my body. I was actually the strong one. The morning after the fear experiment, I woke up with one single lyrical line: *the vanishing path*.

The poet Paul Valéry says that the first line of a poem is like finding a fruit on the ground, and the poet's task is to create the tree from which such a fruit would fall. What was the tree of *the vanishing path*?

• • •

At the end of the first week in Escalante, a day of menacing weather kept me indoors. I watched the gray skies alternate from icy, stinging sleet to snowfall and then back to sleet. Stuck inside, I felt an inexplicable force emanating from the stack of my mother's journals, magnetizing more and more of my curiosity. The gravitational pull of her journals—the ones that I had taken out of the dumpster all those years ago, after she threw them away—became stronger and stronger until I knew that I needed to read them. But in order to do that, I had to call her and come clean first. I was worried that my mom would be angry or feel betrayed. When she answered, I confessed.

"Twenty years ago, I snuck into the dumpster and collected all the journals I could find. And I've been carrying them around since. You're a writer, mom. I couldn't let you toss out your life stories like that."

To my surprise, she started laughing. "You can read them," she said, "but just know that I'm not that person anymore. I purged that anger on the page so that I could be a good mother to you and Garrett. Let me know what you find. If anything inspires you, feel free to use it for a song."

In a moment of shameless self-centeredness, I thumbed through a journal and began reading about my birth. The first thing I learned was that I was *not* born smiling; I was born with the umbilical cord wrapped around my neck, unable to breathe. I wondered whether every person's body has one point of weakness, like a shock absorber for their emotional pain—could this sensitivity be created at birth? Whenever I had experienced sadness, grief, pain, anger, it always concentrated in my throat as a locked-up, about-to-cry feeling. I called her back to discuss the revisionist history.

"Mom, you always say I was born smiling, but I was born with the umbilical cord wrapped around my neck."

"Oh, right!" she said, as though she'd just remembered one more item to buy at the grocery store. "But the doctor unwrapped it and they handed you to me, and *that's* when you smiled." Learning this detail made me wonder what other deeper, unexplored dimensions of the stories I *thought* I knew would be revealed. How many other childhood stories had been painted over with sunshine in the retelling? After we hung up, I dove back into her journals and found the most intimate, truest story of them all: when my mom was pregnant with me, my grandmother Muriel's drinking spiraled out of control.

"She only calls to dump her mountains of pain onto me," my mom wrote. One night, my mom dreamed that she was in a car with Muriel that drove full speed off a dock into a lake. My mom rose to the surface, but Muriel drowned.

"I felt relief at the thought of losing her," my mom wrote upon rising the next day. The dream inspired my mom to give Muriel an ultimatum, and a copy of the letter that is stapled into the pages: "Either you quit booze (with our help—we will pay for treatment) and stay off it, or I will no longer communicate or associate with you in any way. Your drinking makes you violent. I cannot trust you to be around my children. This is your choice. If you want to have a relationship with me or my children, you must be clean and sober."

My mom did not expect a reply. "She'll never do it, but at least I'll never have to face that coward again. Muriel went forty years without talking to her mother, surely I can go that long without talking to mine." Then, to my mom's surprise, Muriel checked into a rehab facility for two months. When she returned, she was a present, gentle mother, someone my mom had never met before.

In her late fifties, Muriel became apologetic, loving, kind. Her spirit was lighter. My mom wrote: "She has a beautiful laugh and laughs often now. She's stopped complaining. She asks all of us about our lives and listens with presence and attention. Every day, she attends either an AA meeting or church."

My mom wrote that Muriel "has become a friend, an ally. She takes pride in her role as a grandmother, choosing gifts and movies and board games that the children love. I even let her babysit! She has said that being part of our family is the greatest joy of her life."

My mom, in 1988, had just given birth to me, and for the first time in her life, she *had* a loving mother. Her happiness glowed off the page. To celebrate six months of Muriel's sobriety, my parents bought her a new car. To celebrate a year of sobriety, they took her to Marco Island in Florida.

In a photograph from that trip, Muriel holds me in her arms while she stands with her shoulders back, looking radiant and proud, as we wade in the clear blue water of the Gulf of Mexico. In another photo, Muriel and I reach over to pet a baby alligator being held by a zoo attendant. The caption my mom wrote says, "Grammy M and Greta were the only ones brave enough to touch the baby alligator!"

My mom described a scene of Muriel stepping out of her car waving, smiling, wearing a flattering new dress, the leaves of autumn at their brightest shade of red around her. "This is the most radiant my mother has ever looked, even more so than when she was a beauty queen. This is the most life she's ever had inside of her."

Then, after fifteen months of sobriety, Muriel died from a heart attack in her sleep. My mom wrote of the shock of seeing Muriel's body in her bed, the skin of her chest blue from burst blood vessels.

"I feel like the Grand Canyon has been carved out of my heart," my mother wrote that day. "She was just beginning to live."

Pouring from the pages of my mother's journal was her true voice—one overflowing with vivid detail, feeling, and poetry, a deep exploration of the maze of her own heart. It was a voice she had confined to the private realm, an intimate, honest voice that never made it into her TV shows or screenplays or novels, which were full of quippy one-liners and rapid-fire monologues à la Aaron Sorkin.

Experiencing the visceral gut punch of her firsthand grief allowed me to see her as more than my mother. My mom wasn't some out-of-touch Pollyanna optimist; she had sunk to the depths of her pain and had written her way back up to the surface.

With this new understanding of my grandmother Muriel's life, I looked back at my familial line again:

My great-grandmother Harriet, lost in grief, was institutionalized and silenced for her pain.
Her daughter, Muriel, found solace in alcohol, to ease the heartache of having an absent mother and an unhappy marriage.

My mom believed that Muriel prayed to the Mother Mary as a way of replacing her flawed earthly mother with a celestial one. That's why "Ave Maria" became Muriel's favorite song.

When Muriel died, my mom played "Ave Maria" on the piano every day, which was what inspired me to learn music. My mother, through her art and healing, built a loving childhood home for me and my brother.

Nurtured by her love, my artistic expressions were encouraged to bloom.

I felt overwhelming gratitude for this line of women, each brave in her own way, each taking strides toward greater expression and a fuller way of living.

What would my great-grandmother think if she witnessed my life? Her emotions had been punished in the worst way possible. But I'd felt safe enough to sing my emotions all over the world.

• • •

Deep in a duffel bag pocket, nestled among clothes and crumpled notebooks and sunscreen bottles, was a bag of psychedelic mushrooms that a friend had gifted me before my Zion trip. "For the desert. In case of emergency," he'd said. I had a vague recollection of hearing that the mycologist Paul Stamets had cured his stutter with psychedelics and scoured the internet to verify it.

In the documentary *Fantastic Fungi*, Stamets recounts his story of overcoming a debilitating stutter through eating psilocybin mushrooms. He accidentally ingested ten times the intended dose, triggering a mind-melting trip. Sitting in a tree during a lightning storm, he chanted, "Stop stuttering now," over and over, attempting to consciously rewire his brain. The following day, he approached the woman he often saw at a coffee shop, someone on whom he'd had a crush. When he greeted her, his voice was clear and steady, and he claims he's never stuttered since. I wondered whether I could heal my voice the same way. I chewed the caps and stems, gnashing the earthy, leathery texture of them between my teeth.

I lay out on the porch in the sun. Although there was still snow on the ground, the day was warm enough for me to be wearing a T-shirt and jeans. When the psilocybin kicked in, geometric patterns began to emerge in the wood of the porch. My eyes were like microscopes, zooming into the atomic level with sharp and clear vision so that I could see individual particles morphing, pulsating with movement. *Oh my god, I can see molecules*, I thought. When I looked at the glass door to the house, my smudged, silvery fingerprints on the door were dancing and pulsating as well.

Feeling overstimulated by the visual experience, I closed my eyes and took deep breaths. I felt a sense of myself diffusing into the world around me. I felt like a cumulus cloud, drifting lazily through the sky. It was a clear day, so I was surprised to hear the sound of thunder. When I heard the thunder again, I realized it was actually the rumbling of my stomach. I touched my face, my arms. *Greta—that's me.*

I float-walked my way to the kitchen craving something decadent. Salt. Fat. Protein. A frittata with caramelized onion. I gathered the ingredients and then I heard that unmistakable voice again. Leonard Cohen was back.

Leonard: Do you really trust yourself with a knife right now?

The collection of his lyrics that I'd taken on my wilderness fast was sitting on the counter, and as I peered closer, I saw that his author photo had once again animated into living, breathing expression.

Greta: Good call. The microwave is safer.

I pulled frozen enchiladas out of the freezer.

Greta: Have you ever tried Amy's frozen enchiladas?
Leonard: I ate nothing but bread and coffee for years.
Greta: A little melted cheese could've done wonders for you.
Leonard: Look, longing is like the grain of sand in the shell. You have to lean in to the grit of it if you want to make a pearl. You have so much longing right now, but you're wasting it.

His face morphed into Einstein's face, then Michelangelo's, then into Barack Obama's, and then back into Leonard's. My body felt like seaweed swaying gently underwater.

Greta: I'm so sick of longing. I wanna be like the Buddhists.

Leonard: The difference between artists and those who aren't artists is that the artists are willing to sit with that longing and to turn that ache into an offering.

The microwave beeped.

Greta and Leonard (together): THE ENCHILADAS!!!

Leonard: What do you long for, other than your lunch?

Greta: A more harmonious world. An end to all this ecocidal madness. I long to stop looking to other people to tell me who I am. I long to feel great love even when I'm not in a partnership. I long to stop trying to escape my body. I want to feel like myself again. I long to heal my voice.

Leonard: So why aren't you using those longings to make an offering? Turn them into art. When you open the shell of your heart one day, do you want to find a pearl or do you want it to be empty?

Greta: The pearl, obviously.

Leonard: Do you remember how you'll get your voice back?

Greta: I have to figure out what to say. But . . . how the hell do I do that without my voice?

With that, the book went cold, his face frozen in a still, black-and-white image. My limbs became heavier as the trip continued, my whole body felt malleable, as though I were made of warm beeswax. The psilocybin acted like a muscle relaxer and I wondered whether this might be similar to the benefit that some SD patients experience with alcohol therapy.

Lying on the lawn chair, looking up at the cloudless, big blue sky, my spirit felt so vast and so mysterious that trying to contain it in one little human identity seemed as silly as trying to shut the sky into a suitcase. I could never sum up my entire spirit into any of the roles I'd played, any of the jobs I'd held, any of the masks I'd worn.

I lay with my eyes closed, feeling the sun's warmth on my face. Every time I opened my eyes and gazed at the sky, my heart felt an endless horizon. It was impossible to *not* be filled with love there—under the warm desert sun, in front of a vast view of the canyon lands. I envisioned a magnetic field that was the collective memory of all the love that had ever existed—the love between parents and children, between kids and pets, between trees and birds, between the ocean and the sky. I was able to touch all of it. I wrote in my journal: *Everyone thinks I am a human woman named Greta Morgan. But, muah, ha, ha, I am an interdimensional love being! But how does an interdimensional love being do normal things? How does an interdimensional love being take the trash out?*

I was desperately and completely in love with everything that caught my eye. The juniper tree—I wanted to marry it. The lizard on stones—I could devote my life to worshipping it.

When I looked at my hand, I was so in love with it that I wrote it a poem:

> Cracked skin like a snake
> Ragged cuticles
> What is that, a beesting?
>> Oh, you are the most beautiful hand
>> I have ever seen!

As I basked in that feeling of unconditional love, I saw a mental image of my body as an hourglass that was pouring all its golden life-force sand back into the earth below me. When the hourglass was empty, when my spirit had dissolved into the ground, when I'd returned to the earth, the source of my life, my spirit, became part of the inner workings of the desert floor. A radiant splendor pulsed through me. It felt like merging back into the current of life that runs through all things. The fear of death lost its bite. In that moment, death seemed to be a kind of ultimate union, the climactic act of a love story between a body and the earth.

As the trip began to fade, as the molecules around me began to go still again, I realized that I'd completely forgotten the task at hand: to heal my neural networks the way Paul Stamets had. I'd meant to heal one part of myself and had inadvertently healed other parts of myself.

In the days that followed, I decided to look for the untold stories of my own life, inspired by my mother's journals. I began, like a detective, to map out the traumas and losses that could be affecting my voice. I'd always prided myself on not having regrets, but as I wrote, I noticed how many times I'd silenced my voice. Why had I let other people tell me how to sing, or to convince me that my voice was too weak, too girlish, too out-of-tune? Why had I been so afraid to express my needs and desires in relationships and courtships? How was I the kind of person who was confident enough to sing to eighteen thousand people but couldn't voice my truth to one bully?

Each of these missed opportunities looked like a wrong turn in a Choose Your Own Adventure story. I wondered if these small, seemingly insignificant moments had had a cumulative effect on the trajectory of my life. Who would I be now if I'd spoken my truth each time I'd had the opportunity to do so?

As my singing voice continued to wobble, a steady voice began to emerge on the page. Each act of writing fostered a new sense of trust in myself and the inner workings of my mind. My psyche felt like a hoarder's den, overflowing with years of accumulated clutter. A giant, tangled pile of thoughts, anxieties, and memories. Each sentence I wrote felt like sending a hand into the pile, excavating a thought or a feeling or a desire, and holding it up to the light. My chaotic emotions slowly gave way to a more coherent understanding.

The more I wrote, the more I discovered the deeper architecture of my own mind—its capacity for exploration, expression, and discovery. Soon, writing on the page offered the same kind of aliveness and emotional release that writing songs had always offered me. The only way to make it through the vocal loss was to write my way through it. Once I began to gather these untold stories, I searched for the meaning in them. Shining the light of understanding on the past seemed to be the only way to build a future without repeating the same negative patterns. As dozens of pages poured out, then hundreds of pages, it felt like Leonard's riddle: *You'll get your voice back when you figure out what to say.*

• • •

My speech therapist, Lori, had told me a peculiar fact about spasmodic dysphonia: patients can often sing or speak without a tremor in a foreign language, since secondary languages are stored in different neural networks. I thought of "Ave Maria" and decided to see whether the muscle-relaxant effect of psychedelic mushrooms would help with singing it.

First thing in the morning with my coffee, I chewed the mushrooms and lay in the sun outside, waiting for that honey-like relaxation to seep through me. I listened to Andrea Bocelli singing "Ave Maria" on my phone on repeat, memorizing the Latin syllables. *Ave Maria, gratia plena . . .*

When my body was deeply relaxed, I listened to him sing and whispered the words. The quieter I was, the less quivering in each word.

Soon, my voice rose from my body. I started recording on my phone. I was "skating" out the syllables on flows of breath. My throat and neck were relaxed. I couldn't believe how smooth the sound was. It was steady and clear, and I felt the calming sensation of bathing in gentle, warm waves.

When I finished the song, my eyes closed, I could feel Muriel's presence on a chair by the window. Every hair on my arms stood. It felt as though she were actually sitting there.

Just then, the doorbell rang and I opened my eyes. The family across the street, the one with the giant Trump flag, had come over to deliver a loaf of bread their daughter had baked that morning.

"We just wanted to welcome you to the neighborhood," they said.

"Are you here alone?" they asked with concern on their faces. *Not if you count my dead grandmother*, I thought.

"Yes, just here for a month," I said.

"Well, honey, give us a knock anytime if you need anything, anything at all," they said, handing me the loaf of bread wrapped in plastic wrap with a curled ribbon.

"I healed my voice!" I exclaimed to Lori in our session the next day. I played her the audio of me singing "Ave Maria." "All it took was psychedelics and my dead grandmother's ghost," I said.

"I admire how experimental you are," Lori said, though there was hesitation in her smile. "Dynamic voice disorders can be affected by everything from stress levels to caffeine intake," she said. "But if you're having a good voice day, let's certainly celebrate that." I could tell she didn't want me to get my hopes up that this could last forever, but I didn't want to believe her. I wanted to believe that I had rewired my brain. My voice was back forever.

Days later, the Vampire Weekend bass player, Chris Baio,

emailed asking me to sing backups on a TV performance. The vocal part was low in my range, would be doubled by another singer, and I'd film remotely, which meant I could do as many takes as I wanted before sending it in so that the production team could splice our individual performances together. Two full doses of mushrooms remained and I trusted that the muscle relaxation effect would happen again. It felt unbelievable to say yes. I was a professional singer again!

The next week, with my recording gear set up, I took the mushrooms, waited for my body to enter that wavelike, warm-honey relaxation state, then recorded the song fifteen times.

There were some little catches and pitch fluctuations, but it was a usable voice. A voice that could carry a melody. After the taping, my throat ached as though I'd been screaming for hours, so I iced it with frozen peas while I edited the best of the takes together. It felt like a great sign of the healing to come. Lifetime diagnosis, my ass. The body *could* do miraculous things!

After my voice recovered from the TV taping, I went to a place called Singing Canyon that Sadie had told me about. It has two-hundred-foot-high walls that create the ideal natural reverb. I stood in the center and sang Joni Mitchell's "Both Sides Now" with more tone and clarity than in the ten months before. Despite some wobbles and glitches, my voice sounded miraculously healthy compared to what I'd been working with lately. I tried to sing my own song, "Other Side of the Boundary," but the highest belting part was still inaccessible. The lower parts of the song sounded smooth. It was such a joyous homecoming, reunited with my voice as though a long-lost best friend had shown up at my door. My body was so alive when I sang, like a fading light bulb suddenly illuminated by a surge of electricity.

The canyon was 10 or 20 degrees colder than it was in the sunshine, so I took breaks to eat apples and almond butter while lying on the roof of my car, then went back in to sing more. When my voice was tiring and my body was cold, I headed back to the house. As I was navigating the narrow curves of scenic Highway 12, a box truck crossed over the center line onto my side of the road. The distracted driver, reaching for something on the passenger side, didn't see me and veered into my lane. I slammed on my brakes, horn blaring, tires screeching, as I stopped suddenly just at the edge of a ravine with no guardrail. The driver jerked back into his lane, barely missing me.

My body flushed with a fight-or-flight response, my blood feeling magma-hot beneath my skin. My knuckles went white, clenched on the wheel, my body rigid as glass. I idled on the side of the road for minutes before my hands stopped trembling. When my mom called me hours later, my voice was choppy again, that awful gravel sound, each word feeling strained, with the terrible catch on the syllables. My voice had become like a lie detector test that revealed any stress fluctuation in my body. I flashed back to all the stories I'd read at the Finnegan Institute office of professional singers retiring because of SD. It made sense now: a singer couldn't book a tour without knowing when they'd have access to a reliable voice.

After I got off the phone with my mom, I took a hot shower

and thought about how I desperately longed to have the kind of mind-over-matter control that some accomplished yogis and spiritual adepts are said to have. Some people's minds are so strong that they can walk across burning coals or submerge themselves in extended ice baths, transcending the limitations of flesh and bone and the subtle reactions of the nervous system.

Accessing my voice and then losing it all over again made me understand my mother's words: *I feel like the Grand Canyon has been carved out of my heart.*

• • •

I began to feel guilty about receiving a paycheck from Vampire Weekend without telling them about my diagnosis. I emailed Ezra and the others to explain what had happened.

"I hope you're all staying positive and testing negative," I began. I explained the illness after our return from Okeechobee, the fact that I hadn't been able to access my voice in about ten months, until the past week. "Perhaps my voice will be able to heal naturally or through injections, and this email will have been pointless, but I also need to tell the truth before too much time passes and it looks like I've been hiding something."

Within hours, everyone responded with loving, kind messages and offered emotional support. Ezra said he was so sorry I'd been dealing with this. "I'm sure we'll send a formal response somewhere down the line," he said, "but for now, just know that we're here for you. If you need help getting in with the best vocal doctors, our team will help you." I assumed there was no way they'd keep me in the lineup. I was the one female singer in the band, and now I could no longer perform those vocal parts.

That night, I dreamed about our Madison Square Garden show. In the dream, instead of performing onstage, I found myself watching the six of my band members from a distant vantage point on the ceiling.

A feeling of finality had come over me. I sensed my time with the band had ended, and accessing a "miraculous healing" felt like a pipe dream. Weeks earlier, a friend had sent me a series of talks by the grief psychologist Francis Weller, but I had bristled against them at the time. Wouldn't grieving be a waste of time if I could figure out how to heal my voice? I'd downloaded the talks but left them in a folder in the farthest corner of my computer desktop with no intention of opening them. Now it felt like it was time. I downloaded the audio onto my phone and headed to the Deer Creek trail in the Escalante wilderness.

My boots crunched the top layer of icy snow as I pressed "play." Francis's voice had a damaged, raspy crackle sound, and he mentioned within the first few minutes that he'd need to take breaks to sip water because of a vocal polyp. I liked him immediately.

"People come to therapy not so much to *fix* what is broken, but to have what is broken *blessed*," Francis said, quoting James Hillman, the father of archetypal psychology. "Wounds and hurts require a blessing from us but we usually extend a curse. Cursing a wound only intensifies it. If we can offer a blessing to our wound, that's when things can begin to change." The wound is whatever forced a person onto a path they would not otherwise have chosen.

"It's not so much that we should be working on the wound," he said, "but that we should let the wound work on us."

I paused the audio to process this *holy shit* moment. Of course I'd been trying to heal my wound. Of course I'd been trying to recover my old voice. I'd never considered that my vocal loss might be trying to heal something in me. I pondered this idea while walking under the stark, naked branches of the cottonwoods and gazed off at the snow-dusted red-rock formations in the distance. *What might the vocal loss be trying to heal in me?*

Maybe it was trying to heal my harsh self-criticism. Maybe it was forcing me to listen to my body, to stop ignoring its check-engine lights and pushing it to the limit. Maybe the vocal loss was trying to heal my sense of self-worth. Without my voice, I would have to value myself because of aspects that will always exist: the quality of my heart, the way I show up for the people I love, the way I listen to the world around me.

Maybe the wound was asking me to heal my sense of hyper-independence, the way I drew inward when in pain, folding my feelings up like paper scraps and shoving them deep in my pockets. Maybe the wound was inviting me back into the wild world. I wouldn't have done the wilderness fast with Sadie if I hadn't been on a precipice, so desperate for insights. The wilderness fast offered access to a kind of love and belonging I hadn't known was possible. I pressed "play" again.

Francis said that when we don't express our grief, it falls into our subconscious but then rises up as depression, anxiety, loneliness. Without grief, we enter a kind of grayscale living in which all the color drains out.

"There's a sacred intimacy between grief and aliveness," he said, "an exchange between what seems unbearable and what is most exquisitely alive." I'd always been afraid that grief could swallow me whole, that it was a gateway into madness, but what Francis said felt like the best pitch for grieving I'd ever heard: Want to access your full aliveness? You better start grieving!

I lay out my camping tarp beneath a stark, barren cottonwood tree and stripped down to my black long johns, which absorbed the warmth of the sun. There were no other footprints in the vast panorama that glowed shades of white snow and limestone. I stripped down more to my bra and underwear and let the sun's rays touch all the soft places on my body. How was a person supposed to consciously begin grieving? No one was going to say 1–2–3 GO and pop a starting pistol.

What was I grieving, exactly? The unreliability of my voice. The fact that for ten months I hadn't been able to sing for pleasure or as a creative outlet. The fact that my body, which had been healthy forever, was suddenly a body that was no longer a perfect machine.

I tried to sing "Other Side of the Boundary," knowing I might not be able to hit the highest part of the chorus:

> *Every time I ever tried*
> *Walking to the edge*
> *My tired heart would compromise*
> *And I would miss my chance*

But I will run now
I will run until I see
The other side of the boundary

Hearing the painful screech of my voice, unable to reach that high register, I felt the ache again. I had thought I would always have access to my voice.

I touched my face—the old tears, the frozen tears, the stale tears, the tears that I was always trying to hold back. My silver camping tarp reflected the sunlight upward. Tears fell onto the mat and collected sunshine, becoming glowing droplets of light. Hundreds of acres of empty canyon land glittered around me under snow. The matrices of hoarfrost ice crystals on the sage bush nearby were starting to thaw and I could hear the gentle crackling of ice.

When the tears subsided, I dressed, gathered my belongings, and headed back toward the car. A tremendous sense of calm washed over me. A spaciousness and lightness filled my body, as though I was taller than when I'd ventured out on that trail. I felt a burst of vitality, as though releasing the grief had freed up all the energy I'd been using to repress it. When I saw my eyes in the rearview mirror, I was shocked by their brightness—green as emeralds, shining, alive.

Before grieving, I'd felt such an intense resistance to this diagnosis that I couldn't fathom having a good life without my voice. After starting to grieve, I felt more open to future possibilities. I wrote down a list of roles I could theoretically perform without a voice: *Photographer. Composer. Web designer.*

Monk. Once new possibilities began to percolate, I decided to dig deeper and research more stories of people who'd experienced life-altering losses. When loved ones had first sent me those hopeful stories of loss and renewal right after the diagnosis, I was in such a state of shock that I couldn't conceive of a new reality without my voice. Now, slowly, my psyche and heart were stretching to hold a wider spectrum of possibilities. I experienced a newfound sense of groundedness and self-trust. There was no clear road map for my life, but I was starting to believe that others, through their challenges, may have left behind some breadcrumbs.

In Mark Matousek's book *When You're Falling, Dive*, I discovered the photographer John Dugdale, who had lost his sight because of a stroke and retinitis and felt so hopeless that he came close to ending his life in the aftermath. Eventually, he figured out how to use a large-format camera and an assistant to make work as the world's first blind photographer. Before his illness, he was a successful commercial photographer, but his work lacked a distinct artistic style. After he lost his sight, the images he created were deep and evocative, pulling me into them like dreamworlds—ethereal portraits of people and places, images inspired by deep memory and personal longing, captured in blue-tinted cyanotype and platinum prints. I thought about how those stunning images wouldn't have existed if not for his illness. According to Dugdale, *vision* is not the same thing as *sight*. Perhaps *voice* is not the same thing as *singing*.

I also read about how the spiritual teacher Ram Dass suffered a stroke that left him unable to talk, walk, or feed himself.

At the time, he'd been writing a book about conscious aging and dying and hadn't known how it would end. During the process of the book, he went from being an able-bodied teacher who traveled all over the world to needing constant physical care, and his ability to speak had been dramatically diminished. In the book, he wrote, "Healing is not the same as curing, after all; healing does not mean going back to the way things were before, but rather allowing what is now to move us closer to God."

I thought that the word *God* could be replaced with any number of things, as though it were a Mad Lib:

> Healing does not mean going back to the way things were before, but rather allowing what is now to move me closer to *my aliveness.*
>
> Healing does not mean going back to the way things were before, but rather allowing what is now to move me closer to *my sense of compassion.*
>
> Healing does not mean going back to the way things were before, but rather allowing what is now to move me closer to *my creativity.*

What if I could allow the pain of what was happening to tenderize and expand my heart, rather than contracting it into a tight ball of resentment and victimhood?

I read about Christopher Reeve, the actor famous for playing Superman. Paralyzed from the neck down after a horseback riding accident, Reeve became an advocate for spinal cord injury research. His story looked almost mythical—an actor who played a hero on television becoming a real-world hero to the community of people who had experienced similar challenges.

In all of these stories, there were the facts of the injury, the medical explanations, the treatments, but there also was a bigger story weaving itself through each person's life.

When I could step out of my own perspective, the story I was living felt like some kind of cosmic dare: a singer whose ambition is the size of Mount Everest sets out to make a swinging-for-the-fences solo record. In response, the universe says, "You want to reach the masses, sweetheart? Let's see you try it without a voice."

I decided to redefine my *voice* as *any expression of my heart.* The way I listened could become my voice. The way I wrote postcards to friends could become my voice. The way I witnessed the world around me could become my voice. The way I picked up trash on hikes could become my voice. Cooking a meal for someone I loved could become my voice. Any art I made, in any medium, could become my voice as long as it came from the truth of my heart.

By that definition, my creativity was boundless.

NINE

YOU'RE GONNA NEED
A LOT MORE TRUTH

ON THE MORNING OF MY THIRTY-THIRD BIRTHDAY, I TOOK A
slice of chocolate cake and a thermos of coffee to the riverbank.
Thirty-three felt symbolic—of beginning a new cycle, of finding
strength. The lunar-solar cycle takes thirty-three years. Gramo-
phone records spin at thirty-three-and-a-third revolutions per
minute. A human spine has thirty-three vertebrae.

I lit a candle and made a wish to the powers that be. "If
you're actually taking my voice, give me something that feels as
good as singing," I said. "Make this a fair trade."

Walking away from the river, I surrendered. I decided that I
would no longer try to control the direction of my healing; instead, I would follow my intuition. A mysterious current seemed
to be beckoning me toward a story far different from the one
I'd imagined myself living. Suddenly, as I was walking the last

stretch of the snowy trail back to the car, the unfinished line I'd been carrying for months completed itself:

> *The life I knew is a vanishing path . . .*
> *No way to move forward, no way to turn back.*

The whole song poured into my notebook as if I were taking dictation. I, Greta, the one who pays her taxes and goes to the grocery store, had disappeared. I became a vessel for the writing to come through.

> *When I opened my mouth*
> *And no song could rise*
> *And the knot in my throat*
> *Could not be untied*
> *I went out searching*
> *Hoping to find*
> *The piece of me out there*
> *The piece that had died*
> *I slept in the canyon*
> *A million stars blazed*
> *The crickets were singing*
> *Their heartbreak refrain*
> *There in that darkness*
> *I could finally hear*
> *The pain in my heart*
> *The sound of my fear*

The life I knew
Is a vanishing path
No way to move forward
No way to turn back
Ave Maria, send me a dream
I know who I was
But not who I will be

For so long I've known
Who I wanted to be
She is brilliant, beloved
Much better than me
There's no way to find her
I know she is gone
So I dance with the ending
As I write a new song
The life I knew
Is a vanishing path
No way to move forward
No way to turn back
Ave Maria, send me a dream
I know who I was
But not who I will be

Days later, I recited the lyrics at Mary's songwriting workshop. "That's what I call a *fuck you* song," Mary said when I finished. "*Fuck you*—I wish I had written that!" She let out a big, warm laugh and the other writers in their little digital Zoom squares were laughing, too.

"I'm worried I'll never sing it, though," I said. "I used to have three octaves and now I can barely hold one steady pitch. I can only sing three or four notes."

Mary said, "Remember when John Prine had throat cancer and he toured anyway? His voice sounded like dog shit but people loved it and they all sang along. You know why? Because he was singing the truth. If you used to be able to sing forty notes and now you have only four notes, you're gonna need a lot more truth in every song." This felt spot-on; I wanted to make that a guidepost for all my future music making.

I was beginning to feel a shift within me. When I'd been dwelling on the vocal loss, my whole life seemed to be crumbling. But now I started to see the loss as a rare chance to build something new. How would I rebuild my sense of identity if I couldn't sing again? Where and how would I put down roots? To what communities did I want to belong? What did I have to offer those communities? How would I support myself financially in this new era? My savings were starting to dwindle, and I knew I'd soon need to figure out a way to earn my livelihood. Wanting to deepen my questions before rushing to answers, I decided to spend a few more months as a Wanderer in the American Southwest. I would listen to my intuition, trusting it above all other voices.

But first, I returned to Los Angeles to pare down my belongings and make space for car camping, to refuel my heart with friendship, and to get vaccinated against COVID. My friends Kyle and Sael hosted an outdoor pizza party for five of our friends to belatedly celebrate my birthday and Valentine's Day. As we waited for them to arrive, Sael gave me flowers signed "With Love, Wyatt and Buckley," who were their two adorable dogs. Sael is a brilliant textile and fashion designer and she teared up when I told her about the vocal diagnosis. "It's so unfair to lose your greatest form of expression. That would be like if I went color-blind," she said. I was moved by her empathy. When they asked about the Botox shots, I joked that I could have the larynx of a nineteen-year-old.

The mood lifted as friends gathered around the picnic table. I asked if the sounds of distant traffic and sirens and airplanes rattled their nerves the way it did for me. "Not at all," Sael said. "You're like a newborn baby," my friend Kevin said.

In honor of Valentine's Day, we launched into our worst horror stories about exes. I loved being reminded what clever storytellers my friends were, what natural comedic timing they had, the way every story ended with a perfect punch line. "Other than constantly cheating on me, Derek was a perfect boyfriend," Clementine said. "My dating mantra used to be 'Expect the Unexpected,'" our friend Thom said.

I shared my technique for getting over one ex, an older man with a PhD in robotics whose only text communication was sending me links to articles or videos he thought I might like. "After we broke up, I renamed him INTERESTING LINKS in my phone and pretended it was a customized news service." I was the only single person at the table. Clementine insisted I should enjoy every moment. "You can eat dinner straight out of the pan, leaning over the counter!" she said.

Before I blew out the candles of a birthday cake, I looked at each of my friends, and making a wish seemed unnecessary. It had been such a good night that my only thought was *Thank you.*

Jenny had moved to Nashville during the pandemic and offered that I could stay at her green and brown Mint Chip house in Studio City. It was strange sitting poolside alone there. No buzz of conversation, no glow of music, no smell of food being prepared. One afternoon during a Zoom session with my new therapist, Shiva, we revisited my past, focusing on moments when I couldn't express myself. We entered into dialogue with my younger self. My eyes were closed as I returned to the scene of my parents' divorce.

Shiva said, "What do you want to say to Little Greta?"

I extended my arm to cradle the shoulder of my invisible eleven-year-old self. "This isn't your fault. It's okay to feel angry and sad and scared."

Shiva said, "Anything else?"

I said, "You are still lovable even if you feel all those things."

A clinking sound brought me back to present time, as I saw that Tony, the pool man, had arrived undetected and was skimming bugs off the water's surface. I lowered my arm and gave him a salute.

Being with my friends was life-affirming, but Los Angeles overwhelmed my nervous system, and I worried that staying could mean slipping back into old habits. I also sensed that it was no longer my permanent home and wanted to search out the next place to put down roots. The vast desert landscapes called to me, since they felt like nature's blank slates. Driving out of Los Angeles, I envisioned myself molting like a cicada, outgrowing and casting off the shell of my former identity and all the expectations other people might have for my life. I would follow Mystery wherever it led.

• • •

The setting sun turned the Panamint mountains gold in Death Valley as I wriggled into my sleeping bag in the back of my hatchback. In the darkness, my headlamp shone like a full moon on the pages of books I'd brought. My psyche felt like a garden bed in which everything had been pulled up and was awaiting new perspectives to be planted. I read for hours, cycling between Toko-pa Turner's *Belonging*, Rebecca Solnit's *A Field Guide to Getting Lost*, and Terry Tempest Williams's *When Women Were Birds*—books that explored lostness and belonging, the illusion of perfection, and finding one's true voice in a world that attempts to drown it out with others' expectations. Each of these writers articulated in a different way something I needed to hear, and I copied in my journal the lines that I wanted to remember:

Toko-pa Turner: "The only antidote to perfectionism is to turn away from every whiff of plastic and gloss and follow our grief, pursue our imperfections, and exaggerate our eccentricities until the things we once sought to hide reveal themselves as our majesty."

Terry Tempest Williams: "Who wants to be a goddess when we can be human? Perfection is a flaw disguised as control."

Rebecca Solnit: "To be lost is to be fully present, and to be fully present is to be capable of being in uncertainty and mystery. One does not get lost but loses oneself, with the implication that it is a conscious choice, a chosen surrender."

Whereas song lyrics used to cycle in my mind, now these new ideas about ways of being, ways of seeing, and ways of creating were weaving through my days. When I was done reading, I turned out my light and gazed at the endless dark bowl of stars shining above me.

The first morning in Death Valley, my camp stove ran out of propane and I went to the Furnace Creek Inn for a hot coffee. As I sat at a picnic table, a dog ran up and licked my legs, which is how I soon met its owner, Avry, and his travel companion, Navote.

They had been best friends in the Israeli Army when they were eighteen but had lost touch when they both married and had families. Avry now lived in Laurel Canyon and worked as a psychologist and Navote lived in Brazil and ran a scuba diving company. They'd just reunited after thirty years apart, to take their two-person flying machine over Artists Palette, a stretch of Death Valley that, because of mineral-rich volcanic deposits, was different shades of sherbet—orange, blue, pink, green, red. Avry played a video of the flying machine on his phone. It resembled the kind of fantastical contraption that a child would invent: a green golf cart fused with a giant, bright rainbow hot-air balloon.

"Do you take adventures like this often?" I asked.

"Oh, this is not an adventure," Avry said. "This is just life."

Navote chimed in and said, "We run the fanciest restaurant in all of Death Valley and all the food at our restaurant is free. Please join us sometime." They dropped a pin on the map where their "restaurant" was, but I couldn't tell if they were joking.

Later that afternoon, I saw it: just off the main road, they'd transformed a flat patch of sandy, desolate desert into a makeshift five-star kitchen. Their camper vans were parked side by side, with a row of coolers and a large picnic table between. Fresh herbs stood in vases on the table, fancy cutlery lay on the counter, and baskets of vegetables rested on bright, colorful cloth. There, they fed anyone who came by, offering all the meals for free.

"Since we are not crowded today, you can be seated right away!" Avry said. "We've just renovated to put in these big French windows." He pointed to the outline of an imaginary wall at the edge of their campsite. Navote pantomimed to an imaginary deck and added, "We have a gorgeous dining patio, as well." They were cracking each other up, and I was delighted to watch them entertain themselves in this comedy duo. Avry pointed at the pistachio shells scattered round their campfire and said, "You'll have to forgive us. The cleaning team was not available to sweep up before your arrival."

Avry made Turkish coffee by grinding whole cardamom pods, then boiling the fresh cardamom with spoonfuls of coffee and brown sugar. He served it cowboy-style, letting the grounds sink to the bottom of the cup rather than filtering it. As we all took the first sip, my eyes lit up with the earthy, caramelized, smoky flavor.

"She likes it!" Avry said.

"I *love* it," I said. Navote prepared tomato and avocado sandwiches seasoned with parsley, olive oil, and sea salt, and when I bit into one, the flavors and textures were so shockingly delicious that I thought, *If all the challenges of my entire life were meant to lead me to this sandwich, it was worth it!*

When I asked Avry and Navote why they'd decided to cook for anyone who wandered by, they explained their upbringing in a kibbutz, an intentional community in Israel where every action serves the collective. "If you're cooking for yourself, you always make enough for another," Avry said. "The secret to happiness is to never eat alone." This reminded me of what my writer friend in Los Angeles had said: "Never lunch alone. Every meal is a chance to network." This was like that, but with the polar opposite intention.

That night, I camped with them and some of their friends at Tecopa Hot Springs. We were joined by Cherish, a woman my age who ran a school in Las Vegas to train showgirls, as well as Cherish's mother, Melissa, a schoolteacher who'd never camped before. Cherish told me that if I ever wanted to train as a showgirl, she could take me from zero to professional in a few months. Now, I could add *showgirl* to my list of voiceless career options.

Avry's friend Scott rolled in on his motorcycle and pulled a giant, golden loaf of home-baked sourdough from the compartment on the back of his bike. Around the campfire, we dipped the bread into an aromatic Moroccan stew. Not only was this the best restaurant in Death Valley, but it was one of the best meals of my life. Scott played "Country Roads," which John Denver made famous, on my guitar. Everyone joined in the chorus: *Country roads, take me home, to the place I belong.* I sang, hesitant at first, my voice strong enough to be heard, yet gentle enough to blend in.

The tremor was barely noticeable beneath everyone's singing along. I had been so shortsighted to think I wouldn't enjoy music if I weren't the one singing lead vocals. Instead, I could bask in the glow of shared songs, rather than be the one in the spotlight.

The next morning, as we all broke bread over a frittata with garlic, ramps, and sautéed spinach, Navote raised a toast: "To Death Valley! Where else in the world would strangers like us gather for a meal?" When we said goodbye, Avry reminded me of his secret to happiness: "Remember, Greta: never eat alone."

After two weeks exploring Nevada, Arizona, and Utah, I headed toward Colorado to check out Orvis Hot Springs, a clothing-optional outdoor hot spring spa that Sadie had suggested. When I arrived, I put on a swimsuit with a robe on top, but when I reached the pool, I saw that everyone was indeed naked—flashes of loose skin, surgical scars, hairy backs, hairy shoulders, strange moles and birthmarks, the gorgeous ballooning belly of a very pregnant woman, surgery lines etched across a man's back. Real human bodies, perfect in all their strangeness. I took off my robe and stood in my swimsuit. *I'll never see these people again*, I thought, and peeled it off.

As I swam toward the spout where the hottest water was flowing, I noticed a man with strawberry blond hair in a ponytail who was reading Brené Brown's *Daring Greatly*. I settled by the waterfall, closed my eyes for a few minutes, and when I opened them, the man was swimming over to me.

"What's your name?" he asked. "You seem interesting."

"What makes you think I'm interesting? Being naked doesn't exactly showcase my personality," I said.

"Your robe looked like it was from a different country," he said. "Figured you were a traveler. Plus, you picked the hottest part of the pool, which means you're a badass."

"Do you read Brené Brown in the hot springs to pick up women?" I asked. No, he said, but reading about vulnerability was what had given him the courage to talk to me. He said that he didn't want to impose on my relaxation, if I preferred not to talk.

"It's okay. We can talk," I said, then opened with my favorite line: "So, how's your whole life been?" He said maybe we should talk about how that year had been, as it had been the first year he was sober.

"What was your drug of choice?" I asked.

"You name it, I used to snort it," he said. He'd played college basketball, but an injury led him to painkillers, which led to harder drugs. His attempts at sobriety always resulted in relapses until he eventually joined a recovery community. Now, he lived in a cabin on the fifty-acre horse farm of his sponsor and he was applying to grad school to study addiction psychology.

When I shared my recent history, his first question was, "Who is your community during this time?" I looked around at the scenery thinking, *Do the mountains count?* "My family and friends love me," I said, "but none of them loved singing the way I did, so they can't really understand what this feels like."

He said that he believed lasting healing can only really happen in community. "Maybe you could join a group of people with voice issues like yours," he said. "Being seen, being vulnerable—it's invaluable in the healing process."

We were both burning up, so we decided to get an iced tea at an outdoor café at the spring. While we sat naked at the table, he asked whether he could write down his phone number for me, suggesting that I should give him a call if I ever wanted to go fly-fishing or horseback riding in Durango. This was the first time I'd ever spent a day naked with someone and *then* gotten their phone number.

When I got back on the road, I kept thinking of what he'd said about how lasting healing can only happen in community. At the St. Elmo Hotel in Ouray, I took out my laptop. I decided to join some dysphonia support groups. I dug into the archives until I found some hopeful stories of people experiencing solid benefits from Botox injections. I watched progress videos to hear the positive changes in people's speaking voices, but I didn't hear anyone singing. Even though my heart felt stronger that spring, my speaking voice had become shakier and more unpredictable, and my speech therapist, Lori, who had originally encouraged me to delay injections as long as possible, had suggested it might be time for Botox.

The combination of Lori's feedback and the positive stories on the dysphonia support group made me feel open to experiment with the Botox injections. I decided that, once this adventure was complete, I'd return to Chicago to try a round of shots.

Around that time, Ezra called me with an offer: Vampire Weekend wanted to keep me in the lineup as a multi-instrumentalist for as long as I enjoyed playing with them. "You bring so much more to the band than just your voice," he told me. He said that they could hire a different backup singer if I couldn't perform my old parts anymore. I felt so appreciated and loved. Some of the old pieces of my life could stay in place after all. The band had just confirmed a festival in San Francisco in October, six months away, and I was excited about the idea of being back onstage with them. After that show, they would begin working on a new album, which could take several years to complete. Their most recent one, *Father of the Bride*, had taken five years, so I knew I needed to find a way to support myself, without a singing voice, during that time.

• • •

Sadie had moved to Moab in the spring of 2021 and invited me to visit and then house-sit while she guided a wilderness trip. Alone in her house, I realized how much I missed the invigorating energy and creative community of Mary's songwriting workshop. My savings were dwindling and I missed working and being of service. Teaching now seemed like a perfect fit. I decided to offer a five-week workshop called the Inspiration Station, all about helping people find the untold stories of their lives, accessing and magnifying their truest voices, and seeking out the songs that only they could write. I announced the class on my social media pages, and to my delight, it sold out.

I cued up a digital jukebox of my favorite records of all time to immerse myself in an exploration of what makes a song great. Listening to these albums felt like reconnecting with long-lost friends. I pored over my favorite haunting folk ballads, dopamine-blasting dance anthems, the triumphant aches of Delta blues, the raw primal energy of punk music. I was hearing the spirit of these songs in a new way, falling back in love with music as a listener.

I settled into a monthlong rental in Santa Fe to teach the class. On the first day, I opened the class by saying, "Worthiness is a gift you give to yourself. Being a *real* artist is something you decide to do." I mentioned Vincent van Gogh, Nick Drake, Emily Dickinson, and Robert Johnson, all artists who never experienced critical or commercial success in their lifetimes.

"These people valued their work even when no one else paid attention," I said. "I dare you to honor your art just as much, even if it's just as an experiment for the next four weeks."

I taught song architecture and composition theory and lyric technique, but emphasized emotional truth above all. "How much did the act of writing a song change you? That will be the measurement of what makes a song good during this class."

The next week, one of the writers, Jade, shared a song she'd written about her brother, who'd died a few weeks earlier in an accident. She sang about how she now counted cigarettes and prayers, making it through each day hour by hour: *Maybe I'll come out of this okay / it's just too soon to say.* Every hair on my arms stood up. She'd used all the tools I'd taught the week before, but the emotional potency of the song had transcended all of them.

Teaching felt like the embodiment of the golden mirror image I'd seen during the wilderness fast: this was a diverse group of people, age eighteen to sixty-five, from wildly different backgrounds, all with different creative strengths, and it was my task to be a reflector, shining a light on their unique gifts and illuminating unexplored possibilities. While teaching the workshop, I noticed that most people miss what's interesting about their lives. Familiarity creates massive blind spots. Like Disneyland employees, we're so entrenched in the daily grind that we lose sight of the wonder people might experience when witnessing something for the first time. We see our plain faces in the mirror. We do our laundry. We spend time with the people we love over and over and over. We take these people and places for granted, entering into an autopilot mode of living. We eat the same meals at the same restaurants. We don't recognize what stories about our lives are worth telling.

Through prompts, I encouraged writers to look at their lives with new eyes, to tune in to their subconscious to access the deeper visions, longings, and desires at work. I encouraged them to find the *a-ha* moment in every song, allowing themselves to be surprised in the act of writing. I encouraged them to maximize their eccentricities, to be bolder in their expressions. I was amazed by the transformation in these writers from the first week to the last. I made a playlist of all the songs written during the class and listened to them, in awe of how many beautiful pieces had been written in that brief time. It felt ironic that the insights I'd gained from losing my voice had prepared me to help other people find theirs.

After the workshop, I went to White Sands, New Mexico, where I watched people ride colorful sleds down the sandy dunes that were as white as powdered sugar. It looked like Christmas morning on the moon. With watercolors I painted on a postcard the white-silver hill with a kid in a red sled and a bright blue pickup truck on the frame. I recalled a funny moment with my friend Samantha. Before she and her boyfriend moved in together, she made a massive list of house rules that included mandatory living room karaoke and legally bound him to joint custody of her fifteen houseplants. My favorite was rule #4: No unreasonable amounts of cheese in the house. On the back of the postcard, I wrote in giant, glittery letters, NO UNREASONABLE AMOUNTS OF CHEESE, and addressed it to her.

For the next batch of postcards, I painted the dunes and added musical notes floating in the air. Years earlier, at a meal with Jenny and some other friends, we had discussed fecal transplants, a procedure where a healthy donor's stool is transferred into the colon of someone with digestive issues. Fecal transplants are often able to cure colitis and other gastrointestinal ailments.

Jenny said, "There was this guy who hated jazz. Then, after

his transplant, he suddenly started loving it. Turns out, his donor was a jazz aficionado."

"Can you imagine just waking up one day and craving jazz out of nowhere?" I asked.

Our friend Jim took on a goofy grin and began bobbing his head to an invisible groove. "Have you guys ever heard John Coltrane? My sweet lord, I love jazz!" He sent us into tizzies of laughter.

"I love jazz!" became the catchphrase that summer. When we reunited weeks later and asked how the others were doing, we all responded, "Oh, I love jazz now. How are you?" "I'm great. I love jazz, too."

I covered the back of these postcards with tiny musical notes and wrote only, I LOVE JAZZ.

This mode of creation felt heart-opening; it was about sparking that direct moment of connection between two people. The desire to create that connection reminded me of singing at my early shows, the mutual recognition that occurs when two strangers feel the same thing at the same time. Without using my voice to build that connection, I'd need to seek out other ways to achieve that same kind of shared magic.

When I was teaching, that had been my voice. On this day in White Sands, painting the postcards and hoping to make my friends laugh was my voice. When I checked into a hotel room in Alamogordo later that night and choreographed a dance in my pajamas before bed, that was my voice. I started to imagine reshaping my life to revolve around teaching, writing stories and songs, and living closer to wilderness. There were so many untold stories of my life, ones that I'd never been able to fit into stanzas of songs, and now I wanted to tell them in new ways.

The second night in White Sands, the park welcomed guests for a midnight bike ride under a full moon. The sand shimmered, catching the lunar light like millions of scattered diamonds. I glided on my bike through the landscape as though I were riding through a dream, the air silky and soft. *This is it*, I thought. *The thing that feels as good as singing.*

• • •

I curved toward Austin, Texas, to visit my brother's family, arriving just in time for my niece's tenth birthday. Garrett, my sister-in-law Bella, and nieces Georgia, who was almost ten, and Gabby, who was almost six, enveloped me in a giant hug as I stepped out of the car in the driveway. Being in their arms felt like standing in the heart of a giant sequoia: they were unwavering, grounded, solid.

Music was on the girls' minds, and within a few hours of my arrival, my nieces and I started a family band called the Gumdrops. Gabby blurted out, "Let's write a song about a goldfish!" Georgia chimed in, "What if he dreams of swimming in the ocean but he's stuck in a little bowl?" Soon, the chorus was born:

> *The little fish,*
> *He had just one wish,*
> *To outgrow his dish!*
> *The little fish,*

He wants to swim
In the ocean blue,
Will the little fish's dream come true?

"What else should we write about?" Gabby asked the moment that song was done.

Georgia said, "Butterflies, rivers, sunshine, dreams, dancing . . . there's too many things to write about!" She closed her eyes and then exclaimed, "What about a song called Summer Sky?"

"Yesssssss!" Gabby cheered, giving two exaggerated thumbs up. Within minutes, she finished the whole chorus:

I was dreaming in the morning light
I was floating in the summer sky
I don't ever wanna say goodbye
Cuz this is the best dream
Flying so high!

I wondered whether the reason kids are so creatively free is because they rarely worry about what will happen after the creation is done. They don't calculate how their ideas will be received or conflate their sense of worth with the last piece of art they made.

Writing was easy, but the trouble began when we started to record. I booted up GarageBand on my computer and plugged in a portable microphone for tracking guitar. Gabby nailed the lead vocals for "Little Fish" in two takes. When it was Georgia's turn to record "Summer Sky," I asked Gabby to pass the mic.

"But I'm the lead singer!" Gabby declared, with the spunk of a miniature Joan Jett.

I said, "Gabby, you're the lead singer for the songs you write, but Georgia will sing lead on the songs *she* wrote."

Gabby said, "But Georgia's not a lead singer. It'd be ridick-a-lous. She wears glasses!"

"What's wrong with glasses?" Georgia asked with an offended shrug.

Once more, I asked Gabby to please pass the mic, but she stormed out in a huff, looking for her mom. I heard her sweet little voice hiccuping through tears in the hallway. "Mama, imagine if you started a band. And you wrote the songs. And then they recorded the songs without you!"

If two kids who hadn't even hit puberty yet could have a VH1 *Behind the Music*–level meltdown over songs about nature, maybe being a lead singer came with an inherent amount of drama. Seeing them argue made the creative tug-of-wars with The Hush Sound seem like an ordinary part of human nature.

At dinner that night, the girls were still ignoring each other. Georgia cut through the tension by asking my brother's cell phone, "Hey Siri, do you know how to . . . poop?"

Siri responded, "I only ingest ones and zeros so I do not poop."

Gabby looked up, now holding back a smile. Georgia said, "Siri, may I please hear you fart?"

Siri said, "Artificial intelligence doesn't fart the way humans do."

Gabby finally broke her silence and said, "But what if you

had fartificial intelligence?" and the girls burst into laughter. The Gumdrops were friends again.

A few days into the visit, Garrett and I tried out his invention, the Neubie, a direct-current electrostimulation machine, on my vocal cords. While I became a singer, my brother became an inventor. After a series of hockey injuries in college, Garrett was told he needed to have open hip surgery in his twenties. At the time, he was studying physics in college and developed the Neubie as an upgrade to early electrostimulation machines he'd encountered at his doctors' offices. Using the machine, he treated himself to alleviate his pain and avoid surgery. Now the Neubie was widely used in sports medicine clinics for training and recovery and in functional medical facilities to treat paraplegia, multiple sclerosis, and other neuromuscular diseases.

Garrett placed Neubie patches on the back and front of my neck to create a microcurrent that was meant to reeducate the communication between nerves and muscles in my throat. With the gently vibrating electrical signals through the patch, I began speech therapy vocal exercises. It felt like a massage on my vocal cords. He offered that I could borrow a Neubie to prepare for the Botox shots and help me recover from them. After the treatment, my throat and larynx felt more relaxed, though I think my brother's love and healing energy and attention might've healed me even more.

While in Austin, I explored the idea of my voice being any expression of my heart. I wove my nieces' hair into elaborate French braids following YouTube tutorials and prepared Moroccan lamb with roasted vegetables, plating it like we were at a fancy restaurant. I continued to write songs with the girls and joined them in their daily drawing and painting sessions. I realized during that time that I'd spent the recent years so focused on building an artistic career that I'd neglected the most central aspect of being an artist—keeping one's heart open and channeling whatever came through. Instead of composing songs, I began to feel like I was *living* songs, and starting to see life itself as the ultimate work of art.

My sister-in-law, Bella, was also a healer—she studies *curanderismo*, the traditional medicine work of her ancestral line in Latin America. The last day I was in Texas, she offered to do a healing, suggesting that Georgia and Gabby could help. Georgia was practicing a tap dance routine and Gabby was watching children's cooking shows on YouTube. I said yes, envisioning a lighthearted family activity, but once I was sprawled out on a blanket outside, the girls became serious about their duties.

Bella burned copal incense. Georgia played a steady, primal rhythm on the drum as Gabby sprinkled herbs over me. The three of them began chanting a haunting, beautiful melody. *Tamborcito tamborcito / ayúdame a cantor / Para que salga la voz*, they sang in Spanish.

Bella placed a circle of obsidian on the center of my throat over my voice box for a blessing, and then she removed it and rolled an egg over my neck, a ritual to collect toxins, sickness, and malevolent spirits.

I felt so loved that tears rolled down from the sides of my eyes onto the blanket under me. I thought of the image of a sound wave, how it is a series of sequential peaks and valleys.

My heart kept whipsawing from the low of losing my voice to the high that my family loved me enough to try to heal me. Up and down, up and down.

Afterward, I had received so much of their love that my heart was like a cup brimming over. Later that day, I looked up the lyrics of the song they'd sung during the ceremony. In it, the singer prays that their voice will rise out and soar to wherever it is needed. "To the heart of my brother, to the heart of my sister . . ." The singer even pleads for their voice to go straight to the heart of the earth. I was unsure if I'd ever sing again, but I knew that I, too, wanted my words to travel wherever they were meant to go.

After two weeks in Texas, I headed back toward Chicago. The Texas backcountry was bursting with wildflowers. As I neared Arkansas, the sun set and the entire sky filled with an electric peach color. I was overcome with a new sensation—a lightness and warmth in my body. *What is this feeling?* I wondered. A champagne energy, an effervescence, a sweetness. It felt new, yet like the most familiar feeling in the world. . . . Then I realized what it was: I felt like myself again.

Not like myself from before the vocal loss and before the pandemic, but like my whole, complete self. The original one who came into this world with all the light, all the curiosity, all the love, all the possibilities. I felt that way without my perfect voice, without a partner, without my dream career, without any of the things I always imagined were the keys to the secret door of happiness.

Somewhere near Texarkana, Dolly Parton's version of "I

Will Always Love You" came on the radio. I turned the dial up and let Dolly carry the lead while my voice fell into the background. I sang with abandon, with joy, feeling the melody reverberating in my body. My voice was still broken, but the person behind it was beginning to heal.

. . .

In June 2021, I settled back into my mom's house in Chicago to try an experimental round of Botox voice injections. For weeks, Lori and I had been practicing new speech therapy exercises to prepare my vocal muscles for the procedure, but I was still nervous and unsure what to expect.

My dad took the day off work to take me to lunch and back to Finnegan Voice Institute for the appointment. Dr. Richardson's demeanor was kind and patient as he explained the procedure. "You'll feel a prick as the needle enters your neck. As I inject the liquid anesthetic, you may feel like you've swallowed a gulp of seawater. It might feel like you're choking, but just keep coughing till your throat clears."

He reached for a syringe of liquid and attached it to a needle. He settled onto a stool, gesturing for me to tilt my head back on a pillow.

"Do you get nervous before shows?" he asked.

"Not as nervous as I am for this," I said.

"Nothing to be nervous about," he said.

Easy for you to say, I thought. *You're the one with the needle.*

"Here comes the pinch," he said and I felt the prick of the

needle enter the front of my neck. My breath hitched at first, and then I instinctively took a slow inhale through my nose to counteract the nervous clenching. "Here comes the cough," he said. The salty, metallic taste of anesthetic chemicals burned my throat, billowing upward through my nasal passages.

"Your neck will soon go numb," he said. "It's concerning for some people because you won't be able to feel yourself breathing. I assure you, you *are* still breathing. You also won't be able to feel yourself swallowing. I assure you, you *are* still able to swallow."

Then he left to prepare the Botox injection. Ten minutes later, he returned with another needle and a small electrode, which he attached to my throat to guide the needle.

I felt pressure on my left vocal cord, then my right one, but I couldn't feel the needle. The actual procedure lasted less than a minute. Afterward, he placed a small piece of gauze on my throat and instructed me to hold it there for a few minutes.

On the way out of the office, neck still numb, I looked in the bathroom mirror and saw one tiny drop of blood gathering in the center of my throat like a tiny ruby. *How strange*, I thought. "Who shot that arrow in your throat?" was the first line from "Wine Red," one of the early songs I wrote while in The Hush Sound.

My dad was waiting on the bench outside the office. "Success?" he asked.

"I feel like I'm not breathing," I said. "It feels so weird."

The numbness in my throat sent a low buzz of panic through my body, and my hands were trembling. My dad suggested that we sit on the bench until the sensation of breath returned and I felt comfortable enough to leave. I listened to the steady drone of the I-88 highway traffic, the soft bubbling of the nearby fountain, the oceanic sound of my breath moving in and out of my nose, the rhythmic thud of my heartbeat in my ears.

"When you were a little girl, you used to leap off the stairs into my arms," my dad said. "You were never afraid of anything. You've always figured out how to land on your feet. It might take some time, but I know you'll do it again."

He reached over to hold my hand. His hand was soft, steady, much bigger than mine. His presence was so comforting at that moment. The idea that I had to win his love one achievement at a time now felt like a lie that I'd been telling myself. Here he was loving me when I couldn't do the thing I was best at. While holding his hand, I wondered how life would change if the injections were successful. Would I recover my former voice? If so, would I move back to Los Angeles, pick up where I had left off on the solo album, return to the same social orbit as before? I knew I no longer wanted to measure my worth by external markers or try to win love through achievement, but how easily could I slip back into those old ways if my voice were suddenly back? Would I book shows right away? And where would I play first? New York, Chicago, Los Angeles?

When we pulled into my mom's driveway, she was waiting outside the front door. "Success?" she asked. Then she asked me to go inside while she talked to my dad. They chatted, her leaning into his car window, for ten minutes.

When she came back in, she said, "I just apologized to your dad for everything I did wrong in our marriage."

"What did *you* do wrong? He's the one who had an affair."

"It wasn't all his fault. Marriage is a two-way street. I . . . I broke the bond first. Before you kids were born. But I felt I made up for it by creating a joyful, loving family life for decades after that."

This inverted everything I thought I knew about their relationship.

"There's so much I never communicated to your dad," she said. "So many ways I could've been more understanding and open."

I was beginning to wonder whether what I perceive of other people's lives is the equivalent of hearing only a few notes of a symphony. Untold stories were everywhere, like dark matter holding the universe together. What else didn't I know about things I *think I know*?

Days later, my dad met me for a bike ride and lunch at a local diner. My voice was reduced to a strained whisper, which Dr. Howard and Lori assured me was normal. It was strange, though, to be inaudible over the restaurant's noise. I figured it was a good opportunity to listen. I typed a question on my phone: "Can you tell me some stories about your life that I've never heard before?"

My dad thought as we nibbled at our omelets and refilled our coffees from the carafe. "When I was nine years old, my parents had their worst fight," he said. "I was used to seeing my mom fall into fits of rage when she was drunk, but this was the first time my dad lost his temper. They were breaking dishes and throwing furniture and then my mom screamed, 'I want a divorce!' . . . and I was so scared. I didn't know what would happen to me." Imagining my father as a frightened little boy filled me with such empathy and overwhelming love for him. He felt his family break apart when he was nine; I had felt it when I was eleven.

• • •

Over the next two weeks, my vocal cords felt wobbly and uneven, like a car with one flat tire. Sometimes my voice sounded breathy, like Minnie Mouse, or Marilyn Monroe singing "Happy Birthday" to John F. Kennedy. Other times it broke unexpectedly like a prepubescent boy's. I couldn't project and my upper registers were still inaccessible. I didn't think I'd be able to sing my own songs live again.

Pandemic lockdown restrictions were lifting and concerts were starting up again, so I decided to post on social media to tell my audience about the strange twist of fate in my life: "As venues reopen and artists begin to tour, i'm not making musical moves the way one might expect," I wrote.

Then, I revealed the diagnosis, saying that sharing it was an important part of my grieving process and of my acceptance, continuing with: "i have hundreds of pages of writing and many sets of lyrics awaiting a voice to sing them. i sense that my new voice, as i continue to discover it, may be fundamentally different from the one i had before. to say that i hope to speak without strain and sing again is the understatement of a lifetime, but i don't yet know my body's timeline."

I clicked "send" and then left my phone behind while I rode

my bike through a nearby forest preserve, taking the same big loops through the Illinois woods that I'd done countless times as a kid. I knew the situation wasn't my fault, but it somehow felt like I'd let everyone down. When I returned from my bike ride, my phone was lit up with three hundred messages.

One person said, "You giving yourself permission to heal and grieve is the permission slip that damn near all of us need."

Another wrote, "You are my favorite artist, but knowing that you're taking care of your body and soul makes me happier than any new music could."

Another said, "Life throws some serious WTF curveballs. May the growth outweigh the challenge."

The responses made me feel loved by my audience as a whole person, not just as the singer who wrote songs they enjoyed. Love was beaming out of my phone screen, and I was actually receiving it, absorbing it into the center of my heart, soaking it into the marrow of my bones.

TEN

THE PURE VOICE

BY EARLY FALL OF 2021, MOST OF MY MUSICIAN FRIENDS WERE back on tour, and I was still searching for a place to put down roots. While my career shift toward teaching was still in its early stages, several of these friends generously offered me their empty homes.

I settled in New York City to experiment with Botox injections from Dr. Andrew Blitzer, the godfather of Botox-in-the-voice-box procedures, the first person who had ever treated spasmodic dysphonia that way, in the 1980s. I felt more prepared this time: the musculature in my neck and around my vocal cords was more relaxed from using my brother's electro stimulation machine regularly, and emotionally I knew what to expect.

Dr. Blitzer did not use anesthesia. He said that I'd feel one needle no matter what, so he may as well just complete the injection as quickly as possible. He tried a slightly higher dosage than my first shot, and as a result, my voice faded to a whisper for almost a month.

Soon, I learned that if you whisper to baristas, they often instinctually whisper back. Trying to socialize was frustrating. At a rooftop film premiere, when I introduced myself to one man, he said, "Oh, I lose my voice all the time, too. You should try chewing gum. It always helps." A friend of a friend said to me, "Whatever happened to your voice, keep it. It's super sexy." While I was eating a salad in Central Park one day, a woman complimented my jacket and asked where it was from. When I answered in a strained whisper, she asked whether I was choking. Her body tensed up, as if she were about to perform the Heimlich maneuver. "Thank you for your concern," I said, and took a few sips of water so that she could see I was okay.

Being in silence made me attune more deeply to the subtle beauty of life around me. In the park, I watched a mother kiss her baby's soft peach-fuzzy head as the child snuggled against her chest. I saw a woman in her eighties strut down the sidewalk wearing a beret, holding a purse shaped like the Eiffel Tower, and sporting a shirt that read I LOVE PARIS. A man on the bench beside me underlined phrases in a book called *Happiness*. The colors around me seemed more intense, the golden yellows and reds of the trees shimmering like sunbeams through stained glass. Listening awakened a kind of pure presence, a more primal and vivid sense of awareness; I saw the world in a way that felt raw and real, without my dizzying, endless inner monologues.

Taking in the scene, I realized that the sacredness of life was always there waiting for me to wake up and notice it, even when I drifted through my hours or days on autopilot. Being voiceless invited me back into the splendor of simply witnessing.

At the three-week mark with no voice, my neurologist's warning that the shots could do more harm than good sent a chill down my spine. I worried it might never come back, even though Dr. Blitzer assured me I just needed to be patient.

Around the four-week mark, I was in the shower shampooing my hair when the chorus of "While My Guitar Gently Weeps" floated into my mind. I whisper-sang, *I don't know why nobody told you / How to unfold your love . . .*

I couldn't believe it: I had more ease and vocal access than I had had in eighteen months, with enough flexibility and control to actually carry a tune. It was a softer, breathier timbre than my former voice, and there was a graininess that reminded me of the rustle of aspen leaves. This voice wasn't the powerful instrument I'd cultivated by my thirties, but there were echoes of my much younger voice—the girlish, whispery tones that had carried my first songs as a teenager. Feeling my voice return to my body reminded me of the moisture within Weeping Rock in Zion Canyon. The water inside the rock provided a life source for the ferns, orchids, and columbines to thrive—and now, my voice was nourishing my whole being from the inside out.

Nearly a year had passed between the diagnosis and the shot that brought a version of my singing voice back. I couldn't help but think that if I'd gone to Dr. Blitzer sooner, I might've been singing with this new voice sooner. But then I would've missed the lessons I learned in that chapter of silence. Through that chapter of writing, solitude, and time in the wild world, I'd tuned in to a clearer, more honest internal voice, which rippled outward on the page, in relationships, and in song.

. . .

A friend recommended the New Voice Studio, a duo of female teachers in Italy known for helping rehabilitate "broken" voices. By that time, I'd relocated up to a short-term rental in the Catskills in New York. On the back porch, overlooking the soft, green mountain range, I logged into Zoom for my first lesson.

The teachers, Lisa and Marianna, wanted me to access my "pure voice," the one I started singing with as a kid before I began imitating anyone else. They asked me to relax deeply while singing, explaining that if a singer's throat is open enough, the listener should be able to actually hear their heartbeat in an elongated tone. Lisa demonstrated that tonal quality by holding a pitch. In the open and grainy sound, the syncopated thrum of her heartbeat was clear.

Marianna asked me to sing simple vowel sounds *Mi may mah mo mu, Ni nay nah no nu.* They suggested that I practice those at night, lying on the pillow, when my body was in a state of total relaxation.

They told me to "dream the note," meaning that I should imagine the sound happening in my mind first, imagine that it already existed, and then just let the note come through my body the same way a dream could come through my consciousness.

This style of singing was all about effortlessness and I began lullabying myself to sleep, the same way I'd learned to write songs in the first place as a teenager.

I spent weeks just learning how to make sound again, to make the instrument of my voice and body resonate. When I was ready for words, I turned to "The Vanishing Path." As we sang it phrase by phrase, Lisa and Marianna kept asking me to sing quieter, quieter, and to peel away all the layers of imitation so I could sound more and more like myself. It was the exact opposite of that Hush Sound recording session so many years earlier. "Pretend there's a baby bird in your hand and you're trying not to wake it," Lisa said.

Once I sang that way, I heard it, and a chill ran up my back, and goose bumps made every hair on my arms stand up straight. It was the way my voice was *meant* to sound. It sounded like the very first Hush Sound recordings before anyone else's ideas about how I should sing had stifled my pure voice.

I didn't have the stamina to sing longer than fifteen minutes at a time, so I sang with this pure voice more like a short daily ceremony than a rigorous practice. This new voice required tenderness, care, and respect. As a songwriter, I would have to behave more like a channeler who could receive a song in one big download and less like an architect who could spend hours and hours reworking the structure by singing it over and over.

Two weeks later, I performed with Vampire Weekend at a music festival in San Francisco. After spending the better half of the year as a quiet witness of the world around me, it was strangely overwhelming to be center stage and to have that many eyes on me.

Since I still couldn't access the top half of my vocal range, we shifted the harmony parts so that Will, the keyboard player, sang my old notes in a falsetto, and I sang his old part in my new, gentle, deep contralto. I didn't have enough strength or tone to perform a solo, but this new version could blend into a layered choir. The backup vocal parts were easy to sing since the phrases lasted ten to fifteen seconds at a time, with long gaps between. Afterward, though, my throat felt as raw as if I'd been screaming. My new voice was precious, like a finite resource. I felt a sense of urgency to record my own songs rather than sing backups.

In March 2022, I booked studio time with Dan Duszynski, my former Gold Motel bandmate, at his studio in Dripping Springs, Texas. I recorded "The Vanishing Path" with my eyes closed, imagining lying on the riverbed of the canyon in Utah where Sadie had taken me. *I slept in the canyon, a million stars blazed, the crickets were singing, their heartbreak refrain . . .*

I used to record ten or twenty vocal takes. This new version of my voice was a much more tender thing, with less stamina. Singing with this unfiltered voice felt like the relief of taking off heels and a tight dress after a fancy event, washing off the makeup and hair spray in a hot shower, and crawling naked into my big, soft bed. It was riveting to no longer be putting on a show of charm or fake perfection, but it was also scary to imagine being seen and heard with that level of vulnerability. I sang the song three times in a row and asked Dan to compile a final version—but there would be no more autotuning, no more nitpicking, no more contorting my voice into unnatural shapes.

When I was done tracking, Dan said it would take him twenty minutes, so I stepped outside into the bright Texas sunshine and watched grasshoppers leaping from the flax-colored grassy hill country, his whole ranch buzzing with the sounds of spring.

Watching the hillside, I thought about the fact that so many of my songs were about loss, breakups, death, grief. *Why*, I wondered, *had I never been able to write a love song?* Not just romantic love songs, but love songs for my friends and family. Love songs for sleeping on the desert floor. Love songs for that lavender color that lingers in the sky after sunset. Love songs for laughter so big your rib cage aches the next day. Love songs for the future. I wanted to write all *those* songs.

Soon, Dan peeked out and asked if I was ready to listen. I followed him into the control room and sat down on the couch. When he pressed "play," I closed my eyes.

> *Ave Maria, send me a dream,*
> *I know who I was*
> *But not who I will be . . .*

This voice, raw and unpolished, felt like a portal to an uncharted territory. Because of the lack of physical stamina, touring and performing my own songs live seemed out of the question, but I was thrilled to imagine recording new songs this way. This voice was meant more for whispering secrets than for belting to an arena. This voice expressed a depth of emotion that my former, flawless voice didn't have.

I found myself thinking about Joni Mitchell, who had rerecorded the song "Both Sides Now" thirty years after her original had been released on the album *Clouds*. Twenty-six-year-old Joni singing *I've looked at life from both sides now . . . / I really don't know life at all* didn't feel nearly as convincing as fifty-six-year-old Joni singing it with the depth of three decades of understanding, her speech smoke-stained, weathered, the voice of a wise elder. Similarly, this version of my voice was a truer outward expression of my inner world, a representation of the previous few years of change, the way the lines of a person's face reflect the history of their life.

I vowed to never imitate another singer again. I was eager to discover what I could say with this new voice that I couldn't have expressed with my former one. If this voice wobbled or broke or went flat or sharp, that would only be an invitation to love it more. Listening back to the song felt like the beginning of a second act.

• • •

What do you get if you play a country song backward? You get your dog back, you get your truck back, you get your girl back.

I adapted that old joke to myself: *What would I get if I played the past two years backward?*

I'd get my house back, I'd get my former voice back, I'd get my old life back.

I thought of all the beauty I'd witnessed, all I learned about healing and listening, the way my inner world had become illuminated again, my friendship with Sadie, my sense of connection to the wild world, and I wondered: *If some cosmic trade were available to get my healthy voice back but lose everything else I've gained since, would I take it?*

The time since I'd lost my voice now seemed more like a string of firsts: The first time I met a stranger on a bicycle who changed my life. The first time I slept alone in a canyon. The first time I spent weeks listening to silence. The first time I understood grief as an access point to aliveness. The first time I saw my parents through new eyes. The first time I wrote anything on the page longer than a diary entry. The first time I sang with my new voice. I valued my voice, all these expressions of my heart, in a way I never had before—as a singer, a writer, a teacher, a human being. I wondered what other firsts would come next.

When a song fades in or out, it's meant to imply that the song goes on forever and that we are hearing only a sliver of it. That's how I've come to think about my life: I faded in from a place I don't remember and will fade out to a place I cannot explain. The task of my time here is to continue discovering the song of my life and to let that song ring through me.

ACKNOWLEDGMENTS

THANK YOU TO MY FAMILY. THANK YOU TO MY MOM, ANNE
Morgan Salpeter, for your unconditional love and lifelong encouragement. Thank you also for generously sharing your personal
journals with me, which deepened the telling of this story. Thank
you to my dad, Alan Salpeter, for putting the Wurlitzer jukebox
in our basement, for being my #1 In Case of Emergency phone
call, and for your unwavering love and support. Thank you to
my brother, Garrett, for being an inspiration in countless ways,
especially in showing me how to turn a wounding into a gift to
offer to others. Thank you to Shelley Gorson, Briana Salpeter,
Gwenny Salpeter, and Gemma Salpeter, for your presence, support, love, and laughter.

Thank you to every listener who has welcomed my songs
into your life. It is a rare and precious gift to be heard.

I am deeply grateful to my editor, Rakesh Satyal, whose empathy, encouragement, and generosity were essential in bringing
this book to life. Thank you to my brilliant and soulful agent,
Alice Whitwham, for making this unbelievable dream come

true. Thank you to Chris Duffy for reading the earliest draft and nudging me to make this story real. Thank you Mark Matousek for your wise teachings, encouragement, and invaluable reflections through the course of writing this book. Thank you to Katia Bachko for your brilliant insights and editorial guidance. Thank you to Natalia Jones and Kenneth Jones for always helping me come home to myself. Thank you to Mary Gauthier and Jaimee Harris for being an evergreen source of musical inspiration to me. Thank you to Anna Lenhardt and Tim White for kindling my early love of language and storytelling.

Thank you to Ezra Koenig, Chris Baio, Chris Tomson, and the entire Vampire Weekend band, Monotone management team, and crew. Thank you to Jenny Lewis for your extraordinary generosity during the writing of this book and for blessing me with your friendship. Thank you to my first musical brothers: Chris Faller, Bob Morris, and Darren Wilson from The Hush Sound. Thank you to all my collaborators in Gold Motel and Springtime Carnivore and to all the incredible crew members who've accompanied us over the years.

I am grateful to my longtime cherished friends, my writing and musical community, and my local Hudson Valley community who supported me through the writing of this book: Sael Bartolucci, Sophia Burton, Will Canzoneri, Hannah Cohen, Lucy Cohen, Myron Cohen, Kathleen Cruger, Kristopher Drummond, Dan Duszynski, Jenny Eliscu, Aaron Espe, Sam Evian, Kyle Flynn, Justin Gage, Bianca Gaiever, Katy Goodman, Elisa Gutierrez, Peggy Haggerty, Misha Handschumacher, Jaclyn Hauser, Rachel Herron, Crawford Hunt, Jim James, Cassandra

Acknowledgments

Jenkins, Brian Robert Jones, Lola Kirke, Becky Levi, James McCrae, Brendan McCusker, Kevin Morby, Donna Morgan, Claire Mulaney, Nirvan Mullick, Eddie O'Keefe, Theodora Portago, Mary Evelyn Pritchard, Garrett Ray, Katie Riggs, Matt Schuessler, Marc Silverstein, Sasha Spielberg, Sophie Strand, Erin Thompson, Sarah West, and Holly Whitaker. Thank you to my incredible Patreon community and all my wonderful students.

Thank you to my voice rehabilitation team: my amazing speech therapist Lori L. Sonnenberg, Dr. Andrew Blitzer, Dr. Brent Richardson, Dr. Steven J. Frucht, and Lisa Paglin and Marianna Brilla from the New Voice Studio. Thank you to Dr. Ryan Hurt at the Mayo Clinic for your work treating long COVID. I couldn't have completed this book without the Mayo Clinic's care.

I wish to acknowledge and honor the Tribal Nations and stewards of the land of Utah. Thank you to the creeks, rivers, and the creatures of the Hudson Valley for being my source of comfort, company, and inspiration during the writing of this book.

Thank you to you, yes, you out there. Thank you for reading this book.

ABOUT THE AUTHOR

GRETA MORGAN is a songwriter and storyteller who has performed internationally as a touring member of Vampire Weekend and fronted the musical projects Springtime Carnivore, Gold Motel, and The Hush Sound. She lives in the Hudson Valley where she enjoys creek swimming and stargazing. *The Lost Voice* is her first book.